Dead People Don't Feel Like Exercising

Dead People Don't Feel Like Exercising

Only Excited People Do!

August E. Mansker

Authors Choice Press
New York Lincoln Shanghai

Dead People Don't Feel Like Exercising
Only Excited People Do!

Authors Choice Press
an imprint of iUniverse, Inc.

For information address:
iUniverse
2021 Pine Lake Road, Suite 100
Lincoln, NE 68512
www.iuniverse.com

ISBN: 0-595-17900-2

Printed in the United States of America

GOD DID NOT MAKE
ANY JUNK!
I BEG YOU TO STOP
TREATING YOUR
BODY LIKE
IT WAS,

PLEASE STOP HURTING
YOURSELF AND YOUR FAMILIES,

YOU ARE BETTER THAN THAT!

Dedication

I dedicate this book to all the children in America.

"Diabetes and obesity are near epidemic levels," says USA Today, January 29, 2001, page 9.

We can refuse to protect ourselves, but we must still protect our innocent children from this danger. If we do not, the problem will only grow worse and their quality of life will be greatly diminished.

Message to a Friend

Okay, so you say to yourself, "I am fat and out of shape. I have tried one million and one diets and have tried exercising to get this weight off, but now I am just bigger than ever."

I believe that the reason you have failed a million and one times is that when you cut your calories you have also reduced your energy.

In addition, when you fight to give up the foods you want, you become exhausted with the emotional resistance and you just give up.

Diets alone do not work. Now, answer this one question, "Can you jump over your house?" Most likely you would ask me if I was crazy. Your answer unquestionably would be, no, certainly not! If I then asked if you could get over it with a ladder, you would answer yes. What I have learned is that we must feed both our emotional and physical energy before we will feel like exercising. It is the mind/body connection. What I will try to teach you is simple, yet effective. It serves as a stepladder to fitness and weight loss success, but remember that you must follow the steps.

In this book I share with you why you do not have the body you want and the reasons you never will until you address two vital ingredients:

— You must stimulate your body from the inside out. You need to flood your body with oxygen to give you more energy, reduce appetite, and expel more carbon dioxide, which better cleanses the body of oxidized fat cells.

— However, nothing will work unless you emotionally connect your six human emotional needs to get yourself in good physical shape. So you find pleasure in the physical fitness process and deeper emotional pain in being overweight and out of shape. Then and only then will you truly enjoy the process and be successful at it.

Preface

I have been in the fitness and weight loss business for over forty-four years. My fitness centers have enrolled over a half million women. When they first joined their enthusiasm was high. Therefore, they got good results.

However, for most that enthusiasm was short lived. When the enthusiasm died so did the hope of being fit, trim, and healthy.

In this workbook I will share with you little known secrets that can bring your emotions, enthusiasm and determination to a near fever pitch. This is the only way most people will ever achieve the goal of fitness and weight loss. If you follow all the principles outlined here, your weight problem will disappear.

A E. Mansker   COPYRIGHT JANUARY 2001

Contents

Forward

The most effective tool I have ever found to reduce a person's appetite is the oxygen stimulator/swish pattern. I used it six times a day to help me lose 50 pounds in five months.

I first heard of it in the Tony Robbins videotape "UNLEASE THE POWER WITHIN" but the concept did not impress me. The only reason I tried it was because I respected Tony Robbins. I was amazed that it worked. Since then I have experimented with various versions.

I preached its benefits for eight years and sometimes got ridicule and people thinking I was crazy. Part of this was caused by the fact that I was not able to explain scientifically why it worked.

Every person except one, who gave it a try, reported it worked because it reduced their appetite, increased energy, reduced stress, and increased their enthusiasm. Many did not follow through because of the fear of appearing silly, or the lack of self-discipline.

Yesterday I received in the mail an article about a study. This came from a professor at the University of Massachusetts at Amherst. It was about the scientific theory stating that hunger is triggered when the bodies' energy resources fall below a set point. This explains why many people's stomachs are full of food and they still feel the need to keep on eating. They are seeking to raise their energy level.

I, like most people, originally believed that we get hungry when our stomach is empty. If low energy causes hunger, lets ask ourselves what creates energy? It is quality nutritious food and oxygen. Most people eat junk food low in nutritional value, but high in calories. What you must have to create energy is oxygen. Most people, who are inactive, especially those that sit a lot have a low intake of oxygen. They do little or no deep breathing.

It takes vigorous physical activity to get a high intake of oxygen. Doing the "oxygen stimulator" six times a day floods the body with oxygen. It stimulates the nervous system by reducing stress and creating an abundance of energy, therefore reducing the appetite. This is only one of its benefits.

What is really great about this is that it costs you nothing to do it. Therefore, I have no financial motive. I am motivated because it will work and help anyone who faithfully uses it.

With hunger being triggered by a decrease in your energy reserve, filling your stomach with junk food is a very short-term answer to hunger. You must have quality nutritious food and focus on getting an abundance of oxygen into your body. This must be done regularly though out the day to prevent your energy level from dropping.

The "oxygen stimulator" is only one useful tool you will find in this workbook that can help you. This book is about my search for over 40 years trying to find a "magic bullet" for fitness and weight loss. It expresses my frustrations, hopes, and also discusses my observations and the many different approaches I have experimented with.

But some people might have given up long ago. I do care about people, animals, art, music, and quality of life. Could I make a difference?.

Like it has been said, "the definition of insanity is to do the same thing over and over and to expect a different outcome each time." Do you have a weight problem? Then try something different. You will have a better chance of succeeding.

I recently sent out hundreds of letters to universities and college professors, asking their opinions about these ideas, along with seeking their own. I got a very positive response.

I recently saw a large advertisement in the newspaper for a weight loss system called Oxycise, which included a book and two videotapes. I decided to order the program and realized that the author had come to many of the same conclusions that I have. We both believe that more oxygen in the body is essential to improve the body's functions, necessary to increase the body's metabolism, and also necessary to experience effective weight loss.

Her book claims a 100% success ratio. But let me define success. To me it means the principles work. Therefore, I can tell you with near certainty that we know how to forever logically solve your weight problem.

It seems that human actions are motivated more by emotions than by logic. Along with the need to gain pleasure and avoid pain, you want to know why you don't have the body you want and why you never will unless you meet or satisfy those emotional needs. We all know that now 95% of those who lose weight eventually gain it all back, plus some within 1 to 2 years.

Recently while conducting a weight loss program, I asked the ladies to tell the group about their problem foods. I asked each lady, and as they began to describe their favorite food, their energy levels rose and rose. If we could only harness their excitement, energy, and enthusiasm, it could light up our whole city. Then I asked them why they wanted to lose weight and the room became very depressed as each one talked about the problems that their extra weight had caused them. They were in conflict because most of the time they only focused on the pleasure they received from food, not the pain it caused.

Each morning I overhear the ladies on the treadmill talk about delicious food as they exercise. Is it any wonder there is a conflict inside of them? On one hand they want to get in shape in order to look and feel better. On the other hand, they feel great pleasure or a distraction in food. Food seems to dominate their thoughts. One key reason is that the food industry spends about one million dollars every hour on advertising using emotional hooks. Does it work? Sure it does, and if it did not then you might not be fat. Would you eat differently? You certainly would!

Recently a disturbed lady came to me complaining about not being able to lose weight from exercising. I tried to encourage her by telling her not to worry about it and that the results would come. I told her to not think of it in terms of 14 weeks, that the benefits from exercising are long term.

Almost in tears she told me that while her husband was eating cheese-cake, he asked her how could she give up cheesecake. Just the way she said it, I knew she would never follow through, and that she would never lose weight or get in shape.

Her attitude made me realize that she was wondering if giving up cheesecake is worth the weight loss. Cheesecake means nothing to me, but it does to her. She was in deep conflict. People in conflict are usually not successful. If it were strongly emotionally satisfying her needs to be in good shape and lose weight, she would not have even considered that question.

Physically fit people are not in conflict. They enjoy exercising because it satisfies their emotional needs in several ways. It is said all people have 6 emotional needs. Yet each of us tries to achieve those needs in different ways. Those needs include: security or certainty, variety, significance, love and connection, personal growth, and contribution.

Those are the same emotional needs that food advertisers use to try to emotionally hook us with in order to sell their junk food. Notice that beer commercials are not about beer but about the emotional hook of significance or connection with friends. Food commercials try to stimulate you emotionally. Their mission is how to connect you with their food. Together they spend over one million dollars every hour on advertising. They would not do this unless it worked for them.

I have developed a series of self-hypnosis audiotapes (Guided Imagery) that a person listens to at night. Each one is for ten days. The first ten days deals with discovering how to emotionally link the need for <u>certainty</u> and <u>security</u> in your life by <u>exercising and watching what you eat.</u>

The next ten days tape deals with self-hypnosis and how to link variety to your life by developing a healthier life style with good nutrition and exercise. The next ten days use hypnosis to focus on significance and how much more significance you would feel by looking and feeling your best. This is repeated for all six emotional needs for ten days, each focusing on connecting pleasure to exercise, eating right, and pain for not doing it. Just like all people who are in great shape naturally do. Does it work? Sure it does!

Some heavy people have tried Self-Hypnosis audiotapes to lose weight. Most tapes were too general to be effective. I found that by directing the self-hypnosis to target one emotional need at a time, then repeating over and over, is much more effective than merely saying that you want to lose weight.

Your next key step is to eliminate much of food advertisers hold on you.

I have developed a videotape to place in your VCR. Each time there is a commercial break when you are watching television, you switch on your VCR for two minutes and watch corresponding messages on the six emotional needs focusing on the pleasures and benefits of a healthier lifestyle. Even the pains of obesity are explored. One way we kill your appetite is to interview extremely obese women about their weight-related physical and emotional problems. Anyone who watches this will deaden their appetite especially for fatty junk food.

The average woman watches four or more hours of television per day. One hour is filled with commercials and half of the commercials are comprised of emotional triggers for food. If you keep watching these I don't believe you will ever lose weight. You and I know you won't quit watching TV. Therefore our Replacement Fitness and Weight Loss Enhancement Videos on linking emotional need to getting and staying in great physical shape and losing weight is the only effective tool I know of to solve your weight problem.

With this you should find pleasure in exercising and eating right. This will support and encourage you. Just ask anyone who has a great body, why they exercise. They will tell you that they enjoy it and that it is good for them. You can do the same and love it! You have also taken a huge step to eliminate the power of food advertisers over you, thus eliminating the conflict in your life.

I believe this is your only chance because you won't change your lifestyle unless you discover a more powerful pleasure in fitness, having a better body full of robust health and vitality. This can eliminate the see saw conflict and put you on the road to success.

Can you lose weight? Sure you can! Can you improve your quality of life? Sure you can, but not by using the same old roadmaps that have led you to being overweight in the past.

Use the new road map outlined in this book and our new fitness/weight loss system. You will experience a whole new journey of vitality, physical and emotional well being. I guarantee it!

Are you frustrated with your weight problem? Sure you are! This book is about discovering what does not work, and showing you what does.

Ambitious Plans

Currently, I am planning to start two new organizations, "Nurses Protecting Children," and "Teachers Protecting Children." "I hope these organizations become national."

Its purpose is to have nurses and teachers committed to fight the growing epidemic of obesity, diabetes and other related health problems that are now a national emergency.

In this book, I have outlined new concepts that are effective in helping motivate people to lose weight and to improve physical fitness.

Nurses and teachers, I believe, have the intelligence, discipline and knowledge to try, test and clearly evaluate the merits of the concepts outlined in this book. Most of these ideas did not originate from me, but are the result of over forty years in the fitness and weight loss field, searching for that "magic bullet," which I did not find, nor has anyone else.

It has been reported that the number of obese people has increased a "startling 57% since 1991." "Diabetes jumped 6.5% in 1998 and rose 6.9% in 1999."

It is my belief that nurses and teachers care about people. They want to help those in need. While most intelligent people know what to do, they just don't do what they know. Some nurses and teachers have weight problems because they overeat to reduce stress and do not exercise enough.

If they are motivated with a strong purpose they can become outstanding role models who can teach and inspire others.

Lack of motivation is the problem. If nurses and teachers can prove to people that tools for self-motivation and stress reduction work then we have a chance to improve the health, fitness and quality of life for many people.

Self-motivation is the key. On the Internet, while searching for obesity related web sites, I found statistics that the entire advertising budget for fruits and vegetables in the United States was less than one million dollars in 1996. That same year McDonalds spent 550 million dollars on advertising and McDonalds is only the "tip of the iceberg". Last year it was said that Coca Cola spent over one billion dollars on advertising. No wonder people eat too much junk food and eat so little healthy fruits and vegetables.

Junk food is a slow poison for you and your children's future and dreams. Our nation's children will be the most effected from obesity problems in the future. We must help them; nurses and teachers can have a major effect.

Sure, adults need to learn effective motivational skills, but for many their greatest motivation can come from the desire to be a positive role model for their children.

Reversing the problems of obesity must be done; our children need to be protected. To be blunt, anyone using their head would know for a parent to feed their children the wrong types and excessive amounts of food is a terrible form of child abuse. It comes both from the parents and the junk food advertisers.

The junk food advertisers are motivated by greed. The parents are motivated by trying to please their children, along with a lack of awareness of the harm they are doing to their children. Remember the old adage, "the road to hell is paved with good intentions." I believe parents should not have children unless they are prepared to properly love and care for them. (If need be parents should be shamed into becoming better role models, only then will their children win.) I want to shock people into action to be motivated to improve their and their childrens quality of life.

In the replies I received from the professors I wrote too, one replied that "the drive to eat is basic, animals will eat themselves to death." He goes on by writing, "culture puts limits how much we should or should not eat."

Television is replacing family and is becoming the force that redefines our cultural values. Since television is supported by advertising, our culture is becoming more and more a society of consumption. Obesity is one of the nasty outcomes.

Do people have the tools to motivate themselves to take control to do what is best for them and their families. This is what book is all about.

Your biggest obstacle to exercise, fitness, health and permanent weight loss is convincing yourself that you are worth the effort.

This workbook is not designed and written for the purpose of entertainment. It is designed to help provide a new perspective and direction for successful weight loss and fitness. I suggest that you do not read over twenty pages a day. This way you can better comprehend and profit from the contents of the book.

It is said repetition is the mother of skill. For that reason, the most important points of this book can be reviewed on different days. This way their value is re-emphasized again and again.

Lets Save Our Children

I believe we live in the most interesting time in history, yet a time plagued with dangers. When I was a child growing up during the cold war, everyone was fearful of being blown up.

There was no television and only a handful of drive-in restaurants existed: McDonalds, Burger King, Wendys', Taco Bell did not exist. People spent a lot more time doing outside activities. Now I realize the irony of the fear of being blown up by the Russians' Atomic bomb. We, have been blown up by McDonalds and other fast food restaurants. In the burger wars, each trying to win the battle, food proportions have gotten larger and larger. Just like trained monkeys, they serve and we eat.

We, the powerless public, are eating more and more which is the problem. Where will this end? If obesity has skyrocketed in the last ten years what will happen in the next ten, twenty or fifty years. Will our brains, determination and body turn into a massive cheeseburger? How much more will our children's health and future be compromised?

It must stop now! My goal is to put together a large group of leaders to organize resistance against unhealthy foods that are being advertised to children.

1. We could try to get the government to spend many millions of dollars on advertising or on government programs to encourage and reward people to eat right and become physically fit. Looking into the future, this is necessary because it could save the billions of dollars now spent on healthcare problems created by obesity.

2. Junk food advertisers spend approximately thirty million dollars a day trying to persuade the public to devour their food. This kind of money would not be spending unless it was effective in getting us to eat more and more. Statistics regarding the increase in obesity are directly related to their increase in spending. The government would need to spend a significant amount to counter balance the efforts of these junk food advertisers.

We need to try to persuade fast food advertisers to cooperate in stopping the psychological attack on children to eat food that is not healthy for them. To appeal to their conscience and if that does not work, to go to the government leaders requesting that they prohibit junk food advertisers to direct their advertisement towards children, just as it was done with smoking and alcohol.

We might not be able to obliterate obesity and excessive junk food advertisements, but we can change the balance. It will most likely take at least ten years to get food advertisers to change the way they conduct business.

When I first opened my fitness center in 1957, the business was in its infancy. It was said then that only one percent of the population joined fitness centers. It took years, but in some areas of the country it is now reported twenty percent are now members of fitness centers.

Personally, I have always been a "maverick". In 1965, I started a mail out to other fitness centers seeking ideas on ways to improve our business and service. Over the next fifteen years hundreds of clubs replied. This resulted in the formation of the National Gym Association, which included over five hundred member clubs. I stopped the association in 1980. To my knowledge it was the first idea exchange trade association of its type. Yet, it was very small and insignificant compared to the number of huge trade organizations in our business today. They have grown because their need grows. Thirty-five years ago, I just was part of the movement that helped light a spark that is now a flame.

As I continue the crusade to fight obesity and to save our children, I do so with a firm belief that it must be done. The time is right and the need exists. My goal is to light a spark along with others to make a change.

During the 1970's, I was lucky enough to start a new fitness system, slashing prices and going for a huge volume. It was a tremendous success that lasted for ten years and might still be going strong today if I had not changed focus. We enrolled over a half million members.

My club's success greatly influenced the fitness industry in California, causing competitors rates to go down as they found that working on a volume was more profitable. Today many clubs charge the same prices as they did twenty or thirty years ago, With inflation counted in, belonging to a fitness center is extremely economical.

In my lifetime, I have seen the power of ideas whose time has come. Believe me there is hope.

Consider This

Does it matter to you that you or your family's weight is getting out of control? Then have the guts to try and change it.

The other night I was watching Joan Lunden on A&E T V channel. She was interviewing former First Lady Betty Ford. The program was about her alcohol & drug abuse clinic.

The cameras showed people going through the rehabilitation program, including interviews, support group, therapy, etc.

Joan London asked Betty Ford. "Why do people relapse and start abusing alcohol and drugs once again?" Betty Ford responded, "hunger, anger, being lonely, being tired that is what triggers a relapse."

I think that ladies quit their diets or give up their fitness and self improvement programs for the same exact reasons.

Everyone knows the standard dieting approach does not work. My goal is to provide a new approach, a new way of thinking that will produce better results.

Lets break down the four reasons for failure. These are the reasons ninety-five percent of people who lose weight gain it all back with-in one or two years.

For over forty years, I have dedicated my time and effort searching for a way to get everyone in the best shape possible. I found nothing works except "you." To get people to be consistent when they feel hungry, angry, lonely, or tired is extremely difficult.

In these pages, I have written about my personal discoveries, why they will always work and how to make them work for you. Give them a try and you will surprise yourself because it only takes a little effort.

It has been said that eighty percent of success in anything is psychological. If you are sincere, then conscientiously start developing the mindset and strategy to enjoy a new lifestyle. Remember nothing will work except "you".

I used the word "FAT" quite often, not to offend, but to make a strong point. Many "OVERWEIGHT WOMEN" try to mentally disassociate themselves from their weight problem. If you keep trying to kid yourself you will never take the necessary steps to get the harmful weight off. A person can be somewhat overweight and still be in good physical shape and not be at a serious health risk, whereas a real "fat" or "obese" person is.

I once heard a very successful person say, "the future belongs to the possibility thinkers, for they will end up with almost everything, while most cynics will end up with nothing." There is an answer to your weight problem, but you will never discover it if you are too cynical to try.

This book is a work in progress. I was just told by someone that a lady started reading this book and threw it down saying, "that I [the author] must have a real mental problem. Fat ladies know that they are fat," in addition to making some other negative comments about me. I am not surprised. It is sad and comical at the same time. Her need to strike out at me was easier than to admit that she needed to solve her weight problem.

Accepting one's weight problem is just like the first critical step to recovery for an alcoholic of publicly admitting being an alcoholic. Not trying to hide or deny the fact, instead admitting to it.

The usual pattern that overweight women often have is trying to forget the pain of their problem by distracting themselves with food, television or some other form of diversion. The biggest fear people have is rejection. Their strongest need is acceptance. You can make yourself proud and remember the first step to conquering your weight problem is to face the fact you have one. Saying, I must lose weight, not I should lose weight. This approach is productive while blaming others is not.

When you choose the behavior, you choose the consequences. You have 3 possible ways to help yourself and your family get in better physical shape to and improve the quality of life.

1. Get the junk food advertisers to quit being so effective in motivating consumers to eat their products. This may not happen because they do not see themselves as the problem. Instead, you

are their prey; they rationalize that they are doing you a favor, a service; because their food is pleasure.

2. Get the government to spend billions on advertising and programs, perhaps even tax credits to motivate you to exercise more and to eat less.

3. You can personally take control and focus on why you and your family are worth the effort.

Now which of these 3 choices do you have the power to influence? The answer is obvious. "You and only you."

Unless you do this every day you will not be effective. Food advertising never quits; they probably spent 20 to 30 million dollars a day, or more, trying to get you to eat more. It does not take a rocket scientist to know that this nibbling at your will, your lack of resistance is profitable for them.

Forty Year Search

For over forty years, I have been obsessed with finding the magic bullet for weight loss and fitness, not so much to discover what works for fitness and weight loss, but how to successfully motivate people to follow through and to be consistent in their efforts to achieve this goal. Motivation is the stumbling block that prevents people from achieving an improved physical fitness and an ideal and healthy weight.

In those forty years, guess how many overweight women I witnessed who watched what they were ate and exercised regularly for ten years. Guess how many overweight, obese women I know who exercised regularly for five years or even one year. Take a guess. Would you be surprised to learn that the answer is "none?" For those who did are called four-letter words like thin, trim or slim. These words are used very often to describe former obese individuals. For it takes the most disgusting of all four-letter words to achieve the trim slim condition. The notorious word is "work."

Let's turn back the hand of time forty years. In 1961, I owned a struggling fitness center on the Square in Independence, Missouri. One faithful day a salesman who I had just hired suggested we run a personal ad in the Kansas City Star newspaper. We placed the ad.

The following morning the phone rang and rang and rang. Overweight ladies would call saying; "I am a fat lady." That fateful day would change my life. For twelve hours a day I would hear the overweight ladies pour out their hearts to me. Each of them promising me that they would change because they would exercise to become thin and would leave their fat days behind.

The original ad read, "Needed 30 Fat Ladies for a new advanced experimental reducing program, all calls kept confidential. Call Mr. Mansker at 555-1212." The ad received a tremendous amount of attention. Placing the ad was both a blessing and a curse for me.

I was married to a beautiful trim wife, yet at night I would go home exhausted and have nightmares about overweight women, echoing their struggles to lose weight. I would hear these stories one after another for ten or twelve hours a day. It would not have been so bad if they "didn't get their hooks in me." If I only could have only detached myself from their problems, however instead my heart went out to these ladies.

Forty years later it still does. Probably no one has ever tried harder to find the magic bullet to help overweight ladies than I. Some would disagree with this statement..

After forty years of searching one thing is sure, I have never found the "magic bullet" to get people slim, trim and fit nor has anyone else. The problem associated with obesity is growing, excuse the pun, "it is huge."

Forty years of testing, writing to thousands of psychologists at our nation's universities, and having several behavioral scientists on my staff trying this and trying that, I found no totally effective formula. With each failure my determination to find an answer only grew stronger.

Success and failure leave clues. In this book I would like to share with you what I have learned. If you are overweight and out of shape, can you change your life? Yes. Will you? Probably not unless you recognize the challenges you face. You will never win the "battle of the bulge" unless you understand your opponent. You can win the losing game if you develop a good strategy and understand what you are fighting.

To win you must learn to think like a martial artist and develop the mental discipline and cunning. You might ask yourself what does fighting have to do with fitness and successfully losing weight?

I believe everything. When I was growing up, I was passive just like many overweight people. Since I was an easy target, every week or so the neighborhood bullies would pick a fight with me, and of course would win.

This went on until a few months after I started working out with weights. Then one day, one of the neighborhood guys started a fight with me. I remember it like it was yesterday. He was winning until I decided I didn't like this and was willing to do something to change it.

After the fight was over there was blood on the ground. Everyone was surprised that it was his and not mine. That was the last of my fighting days in high school. People were more than willing to beat me up, but not if there was a risk it would happen to them. That fight was won by making a decision. "I don't like this."

I opened my first fitness center at eighteen years of age. A couple of months later a friend and myself went to a nightclub. John my friend came up to me and said, "those two guys just spit in my face." I went back and talked to them. One guy said "let's go outside and settle this." Outside I found six other guys who joined those two. Bravely, I told my friend to get back; thank God he did not.

One thing I discovered was that I was not superman. Getting hit with clubs and, beaten badly, I quickly learned that those guys wanted to really hurt us. I was not very successful at stopping them. Suddenly, two guys came to our defense. Now with four against eight our opponents fled.

After it was over, I realized I was not indestructible and I sure did not enjoy getting the "hell beat out of me." I drove my friend to the hospital emergency room. I made the decision for this not to happen again. About that time a new Judo Academy opened two blocks from home. The next day I joined and started taking lessons. Our instructor Dr. Richard Yennie had studied Judo in Japan while in the Army. He was fascinated with the Japanese culture.

His message to us was more than the sport itself. The principle of judo was to get your opponent off balance. In the physical competition you lead your opponent one way then reverse on them. Dr. Yennie spent more time teaching the philosophy of judo and how to use it on a day to day basis.

Everyone has many enemies in life that will hurt you or take advantage of you if you are weak; they prey upon the weak.

I learned everything in business by trial and error. I had no formal business education. Therefore, the principles of Judo were incorporated in my business philosophy.

Soon we started teaching Judo and self-defense in the club. Many of the people I came in contact with taught me street fighting techniques. After becoming interested in weight loss, I read every book I could get my hands on about psychology and conversion.

In martial arts my specialty became the "psychology of fighting." In fighting, the principles I taught were "to get your opponent over-confident and then do the unexpected, attack and finish off. I know I have said this before and I will say it again, "Eighty percent of successes in most things are psychological." Your mindset is critical. Fighting is no different. Since I became involved in the martial arts when I was nineteen, I've never started a fight, never backed down from anyone, and never lost a fight.

Mentally, eighty percent of successful weight loss and fitness is due to a determined psychological mindset. If you are mentally weak without strong determination and a desire to win, nothing will help you. If you are mentally tough, I can teach you how to lose weight, get fit, become happier and healthier. To be the real you

The point I am trying to make is my fight with eight guys is child's play compared to yours, for it only lasted about five minutes.

Your mental and emotional fight with food will last you a lifetime. If you are the average person today you will see daily about 60 tempting food commercials on T V. You will drive past thousands of food signs.

You will have friends urging you to just have a piece of pie or ice cream saying, "it won't hurt you", Just have a bite.

If they are too lazy to get into good shape, then they surely do not want you to succeed and make them look like a failure. It is much easier for them if you fail and stay overweight.

Yes you must mentally fight. You must have a good mental and emotional strategy and stick to it, or you will be beaten up every day of your life.

If you fight back you will feel much better about yourself. Much of life is a war; most of the important battles are fought within you. Decide now not to let food you really do not want or need get the best of you. Refuse to be beaten, refuse to be the victim. Be like all good fighters, learn how to defend yourself then follow through, otherwise you will suffer physically and emotionally.

Fat Is Your Enemy

My friend was telling me his mother-in-law had gained so much weight they had to put her on the operating table with a forklift. She had a serious back operation. Afterwards, in the recovery room she was screaming at everyone because she was in miserable pain. The doctors said that her extra weight aggravated her problems.

The same friend's, sister-in-law at the same time was having her second knee replacement. She is so obese that she has eaten herself into a terrible situation. These are some of the people I am trying to help.

One lady I know is so huge that she is confined to a wheel chair. These are typical obesity problems I have encountered thousands of times over the last forty years.

When I talked to my daughter, who is a nurse in the operating room. I asked her if they ever needed to use a forklift in the operating room. She told me they use mechanical lifts to move extremely heavy people. She started telling me horror stories about obese people she encountered in her nursing career.

She told a story about a woman who was so heavy that when they bathed her they found decayed food in the folds of her fat.

Then she began telling a story about another girl, who while in the hospital was put on a diet. Her mother brought in food for her daughter and hid the food in the large folds of fat on the daughter's body. This was done so that the nurses would not know it. When the daughter was hungry she would lift up the fat and have herself a snack.

For people to have so little control and to be so self-destructive stirs the emotions of both caring and contempt. These people are either mentally weak or have just given up, or both. Just like one of the letters I got from a University about obesity which described some behaviors as "learned helplessness."

Recently, I was appalled when a particular nurse who is a weight loss professional told me about a three-year old obese girl suffering from type II diabetes, when being examined kept begging her mother to get a "happy meal" at McDonalds. The nurse was upset, she said "Something has got to be done," just listen to the power of those words…"Happy Meal." It is really an "unhappy meal."

We then talked about the power of psychological warfare from the junk food industry against our children. She said, "not too many years ago, just about the only type of diabetes in children was hereditary." Now type II is very common in overweight children.

If adults want to destroy themselves, let them. But psychological warfare against our country's small children and conditioning them to overeat is wrong isn't it? No one in their right mind can excuse this attempt at psychological manipulation by junk food advertisers. Just to make a fast buck is unacceptable. You must be totally against it.

I read in USA Today, Monday Oct. 30,2000, Page 8D, about a Scandinavian country where it is unlawful for food advertisers to direct their television advertising towards children. Right on!

This is one of several reasons I wrote to a thousand universities and colleges. I urged them to research how much the food advertising in the media influences the terrible increase in obesity. There must be, I thought some behavioral scientists that believe junk food advertising has an effect on obesity.

Something is going on, one example is on CNN's Money Line Program. They were discussing McDonalds profit is hurting overseas, because of the drop in the value of the Euro currency.

Then they went on to say, "In the 1980's McDonalds average gross sales in America equaled $3.00 for every person in the United States." Last year they averaged $69.00 a person, which is a 23 times increase.

It is true they have doubled the number of stores, and with adjusting for inflation, it still indicates over a six hundred percent growth in sales. How much of a part does advertising play?

Much of the increase has been in the new marketing concepts of so-called value meal combinations, but it is a terrible increase in the volume of fat and calories. It used to be Coke bottles' volume was six point five ounces, now it is often twenty ounces or a "Big Gulp" which is forty-four ounces and a "Double Gulp" which is sixty-four ounces.

What is good for junk food advertisers, is bad for the American People? I believe we should stop this before most peoples' bottoms are broader than the ocean."

The letters to the universities were followed up with letters to the Congressmen, Senators, and State Governors urging this research. Many agreed with me. Is it destructive to be seriously overweight? If you could only talk to the overweight people I have, your heart would go out to them.

Those who are obese eventually will damage their lives pound by pound. Seriously overweight women will have major problems with their body frame. It was not built or designed to support twice the normal amount of weight. It is not if a person will have problems, but when will these problems arise, It is often too late to correct the damage; Yet all this misery and pain can be prevented in most cases; include diabetes, heart trouble, and breathing problems. The old saying "ignorance is bliss" is not helping you become a better physically fit and healthier person.

So far I have not even mentioned appearance. The merits of appearance of being overweight can be subjective, so let us not even go there. Lets focus on health, energy and ones quality of life, Isn't this worth fighting for?

Many people would say, I am overreacting for it is now politically correct to treat people as fragile victims. The big thing now is weight acceptance.

One story we have probably all heard is what will happen if you put a frog in boiling water. They will immediately jump out.

But if you put a frog in normal temperature then turn on the stove's heat, they say the frog will stay in there until it boils to death. This is because the heat rises so gradually that the frog is not sensitive and can't recognize the danger and so it perishes.

Isn't becoming seriously overweight like the story of the frog letting it self boil to death. The danger is so gradual that we don't recognize it until something terrible happens.

Copy of Letters sent

Dr. Andrew Abbott
University of Chicago
1126 E 59th ST
Chicago, IL 60637-1580

Dear Dr. Abbott:

Recently I wrote a letter to a number of universities about the increasing problem of obesity, asking them just how much of an effect that massive media food advertising contributes too impulsive eating while viewers are sitting in front of their TV set.

USA Today newspaper used to list the Nielson Top Ten TV advertisers on Tuesdays, listing the previous weeks biggest advertisers. One week, eight of the Top ten were fast or junk food including: Burger King, McDonald's, Wendy's, Pizza Hut, Pepsi...(enclosed).

One reply I got back from a psychologist at Notre Dame wrote that to get people to develop persistence and to give up pleasure is an extremely difficult task. Maybe part of the difficulty is that the average TV viewer sees about 30 minutes a day of food commercials. These food commercials are using pleasure association techniques to emotionally sell their product.

My question is, do you know of studies on how much this type of massive media advertising triggers increased impulsive eating, emotional or stress eating (not because people are hungry)?

Tobacco advertising has been partially banned because it is considered harmful to the public. Obesity is believed by many health experts to be a bigger problem. Do you know of any such research, or perhaps you know of someone or even yourself that could conduct such testing at your institution. I am not suggesting a ban on food advertising but if an unsuspecting public is put at greater risk because of it, then they have a right to know. I don't have the expertise to do this, maybe you do.

Since 1990 the number of obese people has increased by 50% according to some sources. Since I have been in the Fitness and Weight loss field for over 40 years, neither I nor anyone else has been very successful in helping the seriously overweight permanently get and keep off those extra pounds. I am doing some unscientific testing with overweight women using the theory that most successes or failures in weight loss or fitness is psychological. I believe persistence, drive and pleasure are what we associates pleasure with, even pain. For example, the middle age woman who exercises faithfully and is in great shape loves to work-out. It gives her pleasure. On the other hand, in my 40 years I have never seen one fat woman exercise faithfully for ten years or five years or one year because they hate to exercise. Those that do follow through become trim and fit. Some of my personal story is on the web: www.lifeislikeaturtle.com. The web site for my weight loss experiment is now being set up. I'm also going to write to many government leaders urging them to support government or university research on the relationship between massive media food advertising and obesity. If you know of any research, or have any suggestions please write me.

Sincerely,

November 3, 2000
Congressman Harold E. Ford, Jr.   **Copy of letters sent**
House of Representatives
Washington D C 20515

Dear Sir:

Recently, I wrote to many Behavioral Scientists at over 500 Universities seeking their opinions as to whether the dominance of junk food advertising in the media is contributing to the terrible increase of obesity and health related problems (see enclosure). I have received a number of interesting responses.

I am willing to send you copies of the replies that I have receive from the University's Behavioral Science Departments. To request those copies, write me at:

> Eugene Mansker
> 640 Coors Rd NW Suite. 15
> Albuquerque, NM 87120

Just last week there was an article that the average American eats 300 more calories a day than they did 20 years ago, with less activity which means a considerable weight gain.

For 40 years, I have been in the fitness and weight loss field actively seeking a solution. I have found no effective solution to solve the obesity health problem, nor has anyone else. Quoting Duke University, "the process of adopting a new lifestyle and adhering to it can be more complicated than it seems. Psychological and emotional factors can undermine one's resolve to change."

Junk food advertisers have effectively marketed food not as fuel for our bodies but for emotional pleasure. The average person sees over 30 minutes a day of food commercials. Could Madison Avenue marketing cause the average American to eat 300 more calories a day?

The responses I got back from the Universities encouraged me to write back urging them to do more research on this problem. I urge you to encourage research in this area. If the food advertisers contribute to overeating and health problems, then the public certainly has a right to know so they can better protect themselves. The USA Today, October 30, 2000 edition, page 8D, states "Scandinavian law forbids TV advertising of food to children…"

Sincerely,

Eugene Mansker

Trying To Help
The Overweight

No one has been able to successfully help most people get the extra pounds off and keep them off. The pressures are great, culturally, biologically, and now the mass media is being dominated by the junk food advertisers. I feel this is a psychological warfare against the general public.

In the early 1960s, I read the book by Sergeant titled "Battle for the Mind" it described psychological manipulation and how the principles of conversion takes place in the human mind. In the 1950s, our government became concerned about how brainwashing was used successfully by the North Korean Army against U.S. Soldiers that were prisoners during the Korean War.

During World War II, the Nazis were not able to manipulate or brainwash our soldiers into cooperation, but things changed within a few years. The North Koreans successfully converted many U. S. Soldiers, who were prisoners, to turn against their country.

The book "Battle for the Mind" discussed the psychological principles necessary to get people to believe almost anything.

Religions have been successful in psychological conversion for years.

Japanese Kamikaze pilots during World War II were so psychologically manipulated that they reversed the self-defense instincts for self-preservation. They sacrificed their own lives for a promise of glory in the afterlife.

Today, some Muslims are willing to die in a holy war for the glory of Ala. On television I was watching an interview of a person who was training for a suicide mission against their enemy. During his interview he stated that "in the afterlife he is promised seven mistresses, many wives, great wealth, and will live in a wonderful palace." Most people believe all religious promises are far fetched, except for their own..

"Talk is cheap," yet when something is repeated often enough it causes some people to believe in anything. Notice the food advertising on television and study the psychological aspects. When is the last time you have seen a television commercial featuring fat, obese people? Have you ever seen such a food commercial?

Look at the beer commercials, what do you see? Beautiful people, what is the subliminal message? It certainly is not about beer. No one on the screen is drinking. It is about sex appeal, popularity, friendship, love and adventure. Remember the old cigarette television commercials featuring the rugged Marlboro Man. The individuals' image was strong willed, independent, and portrayed a romantic type cowboy.

This advertising was very successful because it emotionally connected with us, resulting in the selling of many cigarettes.

I remember the first time I tried a cigarette, I thought it tasted terrible. Yet to smoke was supposed to be a sign of manhood, being grown up, and wonderfully independent. Lucky for me, I only smoked for two weeks and thought it a disgusting habit.

This was over forty-five years ago. Things have changed. The smartest people in our society have given up smoking. Why ? Because cigarettes are very destructive. They increase lung cancer, heart disease, and strokes. One reason less people smoke today is because it is not advertised on television. If it were a lot more people would still be addicted.

I bet there would be a lot less overweight people if junk food advertising were not advertised on television.

We are not successful with the problem of obesity. In the last ten years the number of seriously overweight and obese people have doubled.

To be brutally honest only about twenty percent of the population is motivated enough to be committed exercisers. The other eighty percent of the population is not working out on a regular basis. What are the differences between those who do and those who don't exercise?

Just one word "mindset."

What can I say, how can I say it. That is the real dilemma. The last thing most people want to hear is the truth because the truth can hurt ones ego but it has also been said " the truth can set you free."

In Defense Of Fat People

My love hate relationship with overweight   people is frustrating from trying unsuccessfully to help them.

In their defense, the problem is not weakness, but arises from not understanding how to correct the problem, which is not their fault.

Biologically we are in the reverse situation as our ancestors. It is critical to understand this problem because then and only then can we successfully deal with the new problems our ancestors never had to face.

The self-preservation instinct we inherited from our ancestors no longer serves us. In the past ten years the average child is ten pounds heavier. The number of obese adults has increased. In the last ten years we have not changed as a species, but rather our culture has changed.

There is less physical work and more people are spending their hours in front of the TV set. Guess what fifty percent of the commercials are about? Food. Is it about the nutritional merit of the advertisers' food? No. Instead they are using the emotional association of sex appeal, love, friendship, prestige, and being a good parent.

I have heard the average person now eats three hundred more calories a day than they did twenty years ago.

Every TV advertising salesman will tell you the more you advertise the more you sell. Of course, they say this to sell our fitness center advertising on their TV or radio stations. It is true that the more we advertise the more memberships we sell. The problem is for every fitness center ad, the viewer sees over one hundred or more food commercials. If the numbers were reversed I believe many more people would be physically fit and healthy.

"Would everyone?" No. Here is why. Our instincts are inherited from our ancestors. In their world, the main power was muscle power because they preformed manual work every day for many hours.

In their dangerous world they needed to protect themselves by the "fight or flight" instinct against danger. Their impulse was to conserve all the energy they could. Therefore, there is no biological instinct or drive to exercise for exercise sake like there is a biological drive for food. There is, however a desire to conserve energy.

You may disagree with me by using sports as an example, but here is my explanation. Sports original purpose is not exercise for pleasure of exercise, but rather is a social event for the players. The sporting games originated in the training to become warriors for both self-defense and social status. It was essential for survival.

The strongest men were awarded the admiration of their social group, and the admiration and mating with the most attractive females. Sex, prestige, wealth was the motivation, not exercise for exercise's sake.

Through out the entire history of mankind it has always been either feast or famine. Our ancestors were hunters and gatherers. With poor preservation of food, having only primitive hunting tools, food was often scarce. Famine usually occurred every ten years sometimes more, yet fifty miles away, there could be plenty of rainfall and food. Without effective transportation it made no difference.

Hunger is a self-preservation device. It allows us time to find food before we get too weak to hunt for food. Otherwise, our ancestors would have had less of a chance for survival.

Culturally, we celebrate with food. Socially, our main get together is around the table. As a child I remember people saying to me, "clean up your plate there are children starving in China." "As if eating more food would help them, or was it implying that you should have eat all you can now because in the future you might go hungry?

It's is not necessary to exercise for exercise sake. We don't have to physically exercise. Instead we jump into our cars to go someplace and machines do most of the manual labor for us. We sit in front of the boob tube for hours and soak up like a sponge in our mind the sales pitches of food advertisers, increasing our desire to eat. We become a human garbage disposal, making the media and food advertisers rich, while we keep getting fatter and fatter and more miserable.

The average person will digest one hour or more of commercials a day. "We are victims for the battle, for our minds, stomachs and pocketbooks and we are losing."

Overeating does more damage than illegal drugs, alcohol, and ciga-rettes. If we choose to do this harm to ourselves that is our choice and future. It however, is totally unfair to turn our children into human garbage disposals.

What decent or thinking parent would want to increase their child's chance for developing diabetes, heart trouble, breathing problems, knee, joint or back problems, etc.

Can you successfully fight back? Maybe, maybe not, but you should cer-tainly try.

Every decade people are getting heavier and heavier on a skeleton frame that was not designed to carry extreme weight. Nor were our vital organs designed to work with the mass of bulk that the obese are carry-ing around.

How Many Heavy Women Work For Fitness Centers?

Almost fifty percent of the women in the United States are overweight. Because my fitness centers cater to the deconditioned woman, I often try to hire overweight women.

Guess what happens? They lose weight! Being in an atmosphere of fitness, trying to motivate others to exercise and to take better care of themselves is like a powerful mirror reflecting back them.

I was talking to my friend Jerry, who is also in the fitness business, and he stated that, "I don't know many people who work for fitness centers that are fat. They all lose weight."

There are only a couple of exceptions to this. One of my other friends who is now retired from the business had his daughter take over their family fitness center. She is extremely large The other example is a woman who was one of his previous managers, and was the second overweight person I knew in our business. He quickly corrected me that she did lose over twenty pounds after she came to work for him. Upon quitting, he heard that she had put on excessive weight.

In my adult life, I have to a struggle with my weight. The older I get the more I have to watch it. Several years ago, I was out of the fitness business. Retired and traveling most of the time, I would stop at fast food places to eat or to take a break. I began having breathing problems. I was scared because my mother died of lung cancer. I went to the doctor's office. The nurse said step on the scale. I was shocked because the scale read two hundred and forty-two pounds. That was the fattest I had ever been. My former highest weight had been two hundred and twenty five pounds, usually two hundred and ten to two hundred and fifteen was my average weight.

The doctor gave me a check up and everything seemed okay. In the next three and a half months I lost thirty-five pounds. Within five months my weight reduced to one hundred and ninety two pounds. I worked out for eleven months straight before slacking off.

My weight has been up and down. When I actively sell fitness, especially weight loss programs in my clubs, I am motivated to walk my talk. It is the added ingredient that helps me control my weight. I understand how hard it is to stay focused and on track.

The techniques I used worked for me. They helped me lose fifty pounds and was what contributed to my weight loss success. This psychological mindset exercise technique is called the "oxygen stimulator," a combination of mental visualization and physical exercise, including deep breathing.

This does several things simultaneously. First it breaks ones thought pattern and desire for food and promotes energy. It also helps to visualize oneself as fit, trim and in good shape.

Amazingly, this greatly reduced my appetite and relieved stress. Most people do not over eat because they are hungry, but often as a distraction and a stress reducer. Overeating is a habit that can be controlled with effort. The key word is "effort."

Over the last several years I have told a number of people about the "oxygen stimulator." Almost everyone who has tried it has reported outstanding results. It always worked when they used it. The trouble is that most people don't have the discipline and commitment needed to get long-term results, especially when trying something new.

If you are tired of saying, " I am sick of being fat. I want to change my life. The oxygen stimulator works by you doing the mental part so rapidly that it helps destroy your old fat self-image and creates a new slimmer, ideal you. The mental exercises and rapid deep breathing done as described in this book are for 15 to 25 repetitions. .
 If done properly 6 times a day for 30 days, it always works. It tells your brain what you don't want anymore and what you now see yourself as. The rapid physical and mental movement scrambles the old self-concept and sets a new goal. A wonderful, fit, new you!

Searching For
The Magic Bullet

If you do not have the desire or knowledge on how to direct your own emotions and behavior, then by default other forces will control you.

Twenty percent of the population is focused on health and fitness. They exercise and stay in good shape. About eighty percent of the population is focused on food and just sit in front of the television set or computer, and are eating themselves into oblivion.

Some are like my friend's mother in-law and sister-in-law, who are so heavy they are self-destructive. This most likely has been a vicious cycle, making them unhappy. The unhappier they are, the more they eat which serves as a distraction from their sorrow.

My friend is in good shape, which has motivated his wife to get and to stay in good shape. Both his mother-in-law and sister-in-law have destroyed themselves by overeating. His wife exercises and uses common sense in her eating habits. Why? I believe her focus is a result from her environment. Being around health and fitness clubs has provided an awareness and motivation that the other family members lack.

Perhaps her desire to practice what she preaches at the fitness centers motivates her to stay slim. Whatever the reason she is benefiting from it. She does not push herself towards self- destruction by being a couch potato.

If I sound angry, I am; I am just like anyone else who is watching people destroy themselves.

One thing is for certain, it is hard for some people to say "no" to food. The sad part is when someone's life is so empty that food is more powerful than good sense.

Losing weight is a fight, and it has been even for me all my life. I have been able to win the battle so can you. You just need to apply these strategies. Remember most people eat three hundred more calories a day than they ate twenty years ago. Here is a way to eat six hundred less calories a day and to reduce appetite and hunger.

Most people do not overeat because they are hungry, but do so to reduce stress. Dr. Cline wrote me and said, "when you are hurting and feeling blue your favorite food which is so easy and quickly available, takes the edge off that pain. When you are hurting taking care of that is always more important than being concerned about putting on a few ounces." Try these three strategies for ninety days and your life will change.

What 3 strategies?

- Oxygen stimulator
- Mental imaging trimnastics
- Swish pattern

Your Time of Power

Your personal challenge

The power of the "oxygen stimulator" is to remain focused on fitness, health, and feeling joyous. This interrupts negative thoughts, which reduces the desire to eat.

When you think about food, want to reduce stress or want to increase energy, just apply the "oxygen stimulator." When I combined this with the decision to get back into shape, I was motivated to lose 50 pounds and to felt better than I had in years.

Everyone who has tried this technique said that it has worked for them when they used it.

I learned the "swish pattern" from Tony Robins Personal Power Program. I did it to feel better and to be more positive (which is a helpful attribute for sales.) (Swish pattern, oxygen stimulator, & body imaging are all related.)

The happier and more positive a salesperson is the better other people can respond to him. It was not my goal to reduce my appetite, just an outcome. Through out this book I will keep discussing the "swish pattern" (oxygen stimulator & mental imaging trimnastics).

Why Do You Overeat?

It's usually because you are feeling stressed, angry, depressed, or want a distraction.

Why don't you exercise and keep yourself in good shape? Maybe you don't think you are worth the effort or you don't think your effort will be rewarded. Sometimes other concerns may have priority . Perhaps you are feeling negative and depressed about your life. You are in such poor physical shape that when you are around others in better shape than yourself, you feel inferior.

Most likely it is some of the above.

Like many of you I had gained back twenty of the fifty pounds that I had lost. When I began the Tony Robbins new cassette program "The Edge," he suggested that first thing in the morning one should exercise while simultaneously thinking about what you are grateful for in your life.

So I tried it first by using the treadmill thinking about the special moments in my life. I remembered my father and mother when I was growing up. I said out loud "Thank you, thank you," after each good memory. I remembered how my brother has helped me and special moments of my children growing up. I thought about everything that is great in life. On and on I flooded my emotions with great memories and thus, I was grateful. The faster the treadmill was running the more excited I got.

Then I moved on to the stairmaster, I noticed and appreciated all the art-work and the equipment. I said out loud, "this is wonderful, I am so lucky." I moved to the weight machines and by the time the workout was over, I was feeling better, actually I felt great! I was ready to take on the day with more enthusiasm.

Having done this I noticed a huge difference in my attitude. One of the most effective mental exercises I did was "I Like Me," and I thought of all the reasons why I liked myself. My life has been extreme; I have had huge successes combined with huge failures. Often I expect myself to be super human but realize I'm not . In business, I often take on more than I can chew. So I did the mental affirmations exercises saying, "I like me" followed by a reason of why I do.

For instance "I like and appreciate my body because it has served me very well for over sixty-two years. I appreciate the fact that I am rarely sick and each day I am getting in better and in better shape". This gave me a positive feeling which reinforced my desire to exercise. It will do the same for you.

For years I have listened to Tony Robbins tapes and I think he is the very best. Often I have heard him say, "motion creates emotion."
It was not until I started doing the positive mental incantations, and visualizing while exercising that I was surprised to discover that motion really did create emotion.

I had heard about a test using clinically depressed people who were told to put a big smile on their face. Grinning ear-to-ear and changing their posture decreased their depression.

Physically, when people are depressed they have a certain way of standing, with slumped shoulders and looking face down. People who are confident and happy have a more upright posture and different body language

I went out of town and did not work out. On a scale of one to ten my enthusiasm dropped from a number eight to a three. There was an obviously huge difference in my mental state.

The day I started exercising again I was upset with my key employees. Immediately when I started to use the treadmill I did the mental exercises. I thought about all of the cherished thoughts of my family and friends. Then I began emphasizing the good points about my manager and her assistant. At the start it was difficult because I had been focusing on what was irritating me.

While I was exercising on the treadmill I was strongly reaffirming why I appreciate them. In the end, I realized that I was grateful to have such dedicated and caring people on my staff.

Within thirty minutes, I had worked out physically, but more importantly my whole attitude had changed. It was amazing how I went throughout the day excited thinking about what was right and not focusing on my stress.

I found it addictive to feel good. I enjoyed doing Cardio exercises and using weights, while at the same time still remembering all that was good in my life. This has been one of the best things that I have done for myself. I found that combining physical and emotional exercises together was far more inspiring than doing either one by themselves.

Having enrolled over a half million members in my clubs during my lifetime, I have noticed a pattern. The most inspired are the committed exercisers who keep up with their programs, while the uninspired never follow through.

Scientific Theory

For years I have been preaching about the power of the "oxygen stimulator" and the various reasons it works. Most people thought I was crazy.

One of the Professors from the University of Massachusetts sent me an article that I believe explains the scientific theory of why the "oxygen stimulator" works. The theory suggests that physical hunger is triggered when the body's energy resources fall below a set point.

What does it take to create energy? First quality food combined with sufficient oxygen. Most overweight women eat a nutritionally poor quality of food and they don't do enough exercise to get a sufficient oxygen intake. Their energy level is usually below their energy set point. Therefore, they stay hungry. The article says we must anticipate and prevent energy deficits, not merely react to them.

By choosing healthier food and by doing the deep breathing "oxygen stimulator" six times a day 15 to 25 repetitions (quit before you get light headed), you are able to maintain an abundance of energy, and thus your hunger disappears. (If you have high blood pressure, heart trouble or any related problem, check with your doctor before trying the oxygen stimulator.)

The other benefit is the power of goal setting, visualizing yourself as you desire to be. The only way to prove that this strategy works is by proving it to yourself. This also reduces stress, which is a major cause of people overeating.

Energy and Motivation Boosters

It takes 12 minutes a day.

Do these statements make sense?

Oxygen is necessary for energy.	Yes or No
To relax and calm down, ever heard people say "Take a deep breath?"	Yes or No
Laughter is the best medicine because it reduces stress.	Yes or No
Happy people feel less stressed.	Yes or No
Visualization is important for goal setting.	Yes or No
Have you ever heard the suggestion to put a picture of yourself when you were thinner on your refrigerator door?	Yes or No
Have you ever heard of a runner's high?	Yes or No
Fast movements make you feel more alert.	Yes or No

To attract you, food advertisers use happy,
joyous, attractive people in their TV Commercials.   Yes or No

Have you ever heard the saying "A smile is a ray   Yes or No
of sunshine"?

All of the above principles, when combined
together in the right way, become a powerful tool.   Yes or No

---

Ladies weight loss efforts often fail. They get discouraged and gain the weight back, plus some! For those who continue to have a weight problem, their motivation is like the sun, it shines bright, only to constantly disappear, then reappear, and then disappear again. Those extra pounds do the same.

That is why these energy and motivation boosters are so important. They serve
as your ladder to your success. They light up the night so that your motivation shines bright and doesn't disappear like it has in the past.

Discover for yourself. In 8 weeks you will be amazed at the difference something so simple can make. It is necessary however to do your food advertisers log.

Also talk 6 times a day for 5 minutes at a time with a different friend about the benefits and fun of your new lifestyle. This will keep you excited and committed.

OXYGEN STIMULATOR
DONE BY COMBINING 3 STEPS

1ˢᵗ Step… Put your hands on your stomach, then flex your stomach muscles–hold flexed. At the same time, say the word "joyous" so forceful like you are trying to spit 7 miles. This forces you to exhale very hard.

2ⁿᵈ Step… Next reach across your body like you were to pull the rope like on a lawn mower. Jerk up from your hip on the opposite side of arm to your chin, elbow high. Flex all the muscles on your body and say the word "joyous" very rapidly 25 times, each time flexing the muscles. Make sure you don't get too light headed that you will pass out.

3ʳᵈ Step… Visualize a TV screen in the middle of your mind's eye (forehead). In the full picture you are overweight. Place in the bottom corner a picture of yourself thin and trim. Each time you pull up very rapidly, visualize the small picture of your ideal self becoming larger and breaking the screen, and you will see only the ideal you. It's important that you add a huge smile to your face.

Now combine all three steps and do 25 of them very rapidly–6 times a day. It will only take 12 minutes total.

Combining all of these elements will boost your energy and motivational level. Remember don't get so light headed that you will pass out, stop first!

BODY IMAGING TRIMNASTICS

Close your eyes and visualize a picture of yourself. Next bring your palm of your hand from your side and quickly rotate up to your nose- do this very quickly, but stopping right before you hit your nose.

As you do this in your minds eye see the ideal you as you rotated your hands to your face. As you do this say, "I am as fit and trim as Jane Fonda". Repeat this mental exercise 15 to 25 times. See yourself as you are, then as your ideal fit energetic self. This will help change your self image.

Note: You have to be very alert mentally to keep from hitting yourself in the face. which is why this mental exercise is so effective. Repeat 15 or 20 times.

You don't have to use Jane Fonda. It can be someone else who is as fit and attractive as she is.

IT ISN'T A QUESTION OF "IS LIFE WONDERFUL," BUT DO YOU NOTICE HOW WONDERFUL IT IS?

The truth hurts, but it also has been said that "the truth can set you free."

I have interviewed thousands of seriously overweight women in the last forty years. Not only have I talked to the women, I have also observed their behavior.

We live in a world of cause and effect. The food does not jump into a person's mouth. A decision was made to put it there. Why is it easier for the thin woman to say "no" to food than for the overweight woman. What are the psychological differences?

Certainly, there is more than one reason One is the overweight lady may feel more isolated and alone. She turns to food for comfort, and to fill up the emptiness. Naturally, the degrees of this will vary from individual to individual. Again, it has been reported that many people overeat to reduce stress.

Happy, optimistic people are generally more outgoing and actively take better care of themselves. People do not become extremely overweight overnight. It is achieved over a period of years. A couple hundred extra calories a day can generate a different outcome of forty or fifty pounds, even two hundred pounds!

Emotionally, feeling good about oneself and one's future can make a huge difference. A moderate amount of exercise can produce meaningful benefits.

Consistency is extremely important. Can you guess in the last forty years how many heavy women I have known who exercised regularly for ten years? For five years? For even one year? Again, the answer is none. Those that did were called four letter words, "trim," "thin," and "slim."

I have heard so many fat women make promises saying, "I am going to get this weight off and keep it off." For years I have believed them. but now I just sincerely hope they will follow though.

"Excuses are like your heart, everyone has got one." Even outside my business when I meet women and tell them what I do for a living, many will say " I used to go to a gym, but I quit because this or that thing was wrong with them."

They blamed the fitness center for them quitting. They never admitted that it was just too much work, or that they were just too lazy.

Women who join my fitness center sign a membership contract to pay for a certain period of time. When they get behind on their payments we call them. Most will always have an excuse, often blaming us. "There is something wrong with us, never them."

Most are fun to be around, yet a few who do not get their own way are experts at making every ones' life miserable.

The point of all this is not to criticize, but to point out the value and need for a person to feel grateful for their life. You should cherish yourself and most of all appreciate your own body. If you hate your body, how can you love yourself?

If you do not appreciate your body, your self worth suffers. Is it worth making the effort? Instead, you could turn to food to distract you from the pain of life.

Television, radio & newspaper advertisers spend billions of dollars every year to get you to emotionally focus on food. Restaurants are everywhere and fitness centers are not.

If you do not want junk food advertisers to direct your mind then you must take control. You must conscientiously develop the desire to improve and reinforce the desire everyday for at least thirty minutes. Most likely you will see thirty minutes a day of food commercials trying to encourage you to eat, to gain weight and to become fat.

Eighty percent of success is psychological, so develop a strong mind-set to be happy, to be fit, and to be successful.

This Always Works, When You Do!

Now you can have the body you deserve, these one hundred ladies tried the oxygen stimulators and it worked for them and it can work for you.

One demonstration we showed the ladies before they tried the oxygen stimulator was lighting a candle, then placing a glass directly over it. Guess what happened? Within three to five seconds the flame went out. Why? Because nothing can burn without oxygen.

Remember the old type fireplace bellows that were used to start fires in the wood or coal fireplaces, (even blacksmiths had them). You hand pumps them very rapidly holding it close to the flame. The extra air helped start the fire.

The demonstration helped remind the ladies that nothing will burn without oxygen including body fat. The more oxygen you get the faster things burn, even body fat! If your lungs hold up to two gallons of air and you breathe only two pints, then you lack sufficient oxygen to create massive energy. If you don't have an abundance of energy then you don't feel like doing much including exercising.

One hundred percent of these women surveyed said the oxygen stimulator helped them to increase energy, reduce stress or reduce appetite.

Johanna Rondeau
KoriAnn Sanchez
Carla Jio
Karen Hernandez
Geneva Padilla
Liz Johnson
Belva Butterfield
Belinda Hall
Deidre Wilkerson
Helen Lisle
Sheila Husman
Meri Lee
Terri Fragua
Faye Hansen
Janet Gillett
Barbara Gillett
Henrietta Zamarron
Renee O'Donnell
Matida Mayo
Monica Hilaljo
Alissa Cardova
Marlene Morrish
Rachel Hix
Debbie Bolling
Raelene Almaguer
Patti Hager
Rachel Bande

Margaret Sando
Bridgett Phillips

Margaret Pancho
Yolanda Garcia
Renee Ymumoz
Candy Bennett
Debbie Sanchez
Jackie DeVincentis
Nicole MeyersConsuelo
Beverly Chavez
Namomi Burgos-Loesch
Julia Ann Gacia
Robin Miller
Mari Jo Vigil
JaJa Goetz
Mary Campos
Cindy Martinez
Lynette Montoya
Deidre Willherson

This is only a few of the women who have had positive results. It always works when you do! In five years only two women told me it did not work, I believe the reason was they were not doing it right.

Breathing is your first act when you are born. You take a deep breath, and when you die, you let it out, this is your last act. How deep you breathe will help determine how much energy you have all during your life.

The more energy you have the more you want to do! Simple but true.

Anyone Can Lose
Weight And Most Do

Almost everyone, when they are motivated and exercise regularly, achieve good results. Losing weight is simple, just take in fewer calories than your body burns up.

The problem is not that people do not make progress, it is solely because their efforts cease. They revert back to their old bad habits. If they lose weight they gain it all back, plus more.

I have met a large number of seriously overweight women who have told me they had reached their ideal weight before. Some, more than once gained it all back. I think there are several reasons for this. One reason is I think many overweight women fantasize that when they lose weight, all of a sudden their problems will disappear. Their life will be perfect. Another reason is a crisis may appear in their lives while they are trying to lose weight. This crisis puts them under a lot of stress. Sometimes it is so demanding of their focus, their weight loss or fitness ceases to be a priority. In short, what motivated them to make the effort to lose weight and improve themselves has lost its power.

If you say to most people eighty percent of success in weight loss is psychological they would swear we are mentally nuts. Calories, from food, are what puts the weight on you.

I say, yes you are right, but food does not jump into your mouth. Your mindset determines what and how much food you put into your mouth. Even what foods you like. Your mindset determines if you enjoy the activity of exercise even if you enjoy the process of losing weight and getting fit.

If the process is not enjoyable to you, then most likely you will never follow through and you will never lose weight nor stay fit.

I challenge anyone to dispute this fact and prove me wrong. The only exception is when a person does hard manual labor for a living. They might hate it, but they don't have a weight problem.

Heredity does not cause most people to be over-weight. I heard a big nurse say, "genetics caused her weight problem." She got violently mad when I disagreed with her. I told her my grandfather weighed over three hundred pounds and all my family was overweight from time to time including myself. Yet, when I do the right things the extra weight comes off. Almost everyone I know who is in good shape also has fat unmotivated relatives.

Most people do not want to hear the truth. They do not want to take responsibility for their own lives. Yet, if they do not they will pay the price and suffer the pain, not if, but when.

Forty years ago, when I first started trying to help overweight women conquer their weight problem, there was one woman I will never forget. I was interviewing her. After a few minutes she broke into tears sobbing as she relayed what had happened to her that morning. Her husband had awakened, rolled over and stared at her and said "I wonder what it would be like to make love to a slender woman just once." I tried to comfort her, She promised me that she would lose eighty pounds and that she would clean herself up and be neater. She even wrote a check and paid in full for one year.

Back then memberships were more expensive than they are today. We set her an appointment that she did not keep. I sincerely wanted to help this lady. It was not until two weeks later when I reached her by telephone.

I asked her how was she doing and if she would like to set up a time to get started. Her reply shocked me "Oh everything is okay, my husband apologized and said he did not mean it." I asked her when could we get you started on your weight loss and exercise program? She said, "Oh I don't care about that now."

Over the years I have often told this story. Everyone agrees her husband did mean it, but she probably made him feel guilty so that he apologized.

Around the fitness centers they say the only type of man who wants a seriously overweight woman is a very insecure man. I have heard many unhappy men around the gyms say thousands of times that their wives were in good shape when they got married and then grew heavy. The men grew numb to it, but they didn't like it. I have never heard one man say, "I want a really fat woman."

Over the years, I have heard many women who called the clubs saying that their husbands gave them the phone number for our weight loss program. It is the husbands, sometimes who have their wives call us.

For example, a woman had gained sixty pounds since she and her husband had gotten married. She started crying and said to her husband that he should accept her the way she was. Life is an effort. Are you worth the effort? Or do you think that pleasing your husband is worth the effort?

Now make a list of all your old favorite excuses for not exercising or losing weight.

Now make another list of all the reasons you want to get in shape, lose weight, and enjoy the process.

On Duke
University's Website

A life style change is more difficult than most people think. The process of adapting a new lifestyle and adhering to it can be more complicated than it seems. Psychological and emotional factors can undermine one's resolve to change.

I know you have read this before, but do you have the will to fight? Losing weight is a fight. It always has been for many of us. If you do not know how to fight, then you shall be beaten.

Like I wrote when I was a young boy, I was passive and the more aggressive neighborhood boys used me regularly as a punching bag. Emotionally humiliated, I pulled into my shell.

When I started working out with weights, things changed. I won the next fight because I decided to. That was my last fight in school. The guy I beat was a tough guy so my former opponents decided not to take any chances.

We taught "Judo & Self-Defense" in our fitness center. Members of the police force joined to learn self-defense. At this time, I became interested in psychology, reading hundreds of books on the subject. One of my main interests became the "psychological principles of fighting."

I would later teach these. The first step is to get your opponent over confident. People are basically lazy and will usually exert only the effort they believe necessary to win. If they think you are easy they are more likely to be careless. Second, do the "unexpected," this confuses them and gives you the element of surprise. Third, is to attack and last, quickly finish off your opponent by putting him out of commission. Otherwise, they can recover and beat the hell out of you.

Fighting is a very serious thing. The best fight you ever win is the one you stay out of.

Eighty percent of success in most things is psychological. Let's again examine the psychology of my fighting. When I was young, I was beaten and humiliated constantly. This put me in psychological pain. I thought of myself as a loser and as a result, inferior. The psychological pain hurt more than the physical.

Over the years, I have been in a few fights, far less than when I was young and an easy target. I try to avoid being in a situation, but I am in the business around a lot of physical hotheads.

In most cases, doing the unexpected and breaking your opponents' confidence causes them to back down. Then the fight is over, and no one is hurt. Yet, a person's pride is undamaged.

I know many women who think fighting is terrible. I believe the same, but sometimes you do not have a choice. Being willing to fight is most of the battle. You would not let someone attack and hurt your family while just standing back, would you? Get mad, get determined! What is your enemy? Junk food!

If you are mentally or emotionally weak you must change! Not should, but must!

You Must Exercise!

Many women feel that cutting caloric intake is enough to lose weight. Sure you can take off pounds but that does not insure you will look and really feel in shape. You can have a lot of flab or loose skin hanging everywhere on your body. Many women who lose weight at simply counting calories look worse than they did before.
You can spend twenty to fifty thousand to have your stomach stapled. I have meet several women who have busted out the staples. I have heard a doctor say, "about twenty percent of the time staples break or the stomach stretches and expands which causes the operation to fail". I have seen many women who have had the operation only to look like death warmed over.

You can have liposuction and end up gaining the unwanted fat back.. You need to exercise to firm up, to improve your posture, look better and be healthy.

Joining a fitness center is the best way to get in shape, providing you choose the right one. Years ago there were few fitness centers and they catered to everybody. Now there are several types.

Here are some suggestions. Choose a fitness club where you will not feel out of place. Many women tell me they joined a co-ed club and disliked it for these reasons.

- They were older and the fitness center members were young and in great shape.

- The older or overweight felt as if they were a locker room joke. Many over-heard unpleasant comments.

- The staff was young and spent their time flirting with each other and the young attractive members, ignoring every one else. In short the co-ed clubs is a meat market or meet market.

- The younger more attractive women felt uncomfortable with the unwanted looks and advances.

- The women said their husband did not like them going to a co-ed fitness center.

All of the above reasons are true. When I visit fitness clubs I count the percentage of people less than thirty years of age, and over thirty. In most cases in the exercise classes 90% percent are under thirty. I also count the number of overweight or obese women. Again it is about ten percent and about zero for the obese.

Some women join gyms or co-ed fitness centers but they feel uncomfortable as well as not being able to keep up so they drop out and stop going. I can relate to this, I was sixteen years old when I joined my first gym. Now I am in my mid sixties. Back then I wanted to workout with guys who were my age. We competed to see "who could lift the most weight, who had the biggest biceps or chest Now fifty years later I am not as strong and well built, with human nature being as it is I do not want to look in the gyms mirrors standing next to twenty year old muscles men and to be reminded constantly that I am older and slipping physically. I do not want to feel physically inferior and if you are completely honest, neither do you.

In short, choose a fitness center that caters to people like you. This will cause you to feel more comfortable and therefore use the club more, giving you greater results.

Ask yourself, what do I want to accomplish? Why do I want to achieve this? Look at the club members and ask yourself will I feel comfortable here? If you are self conscious about your weight or age you would most likely feel out of place in at a gym or most co-ed fitness centers.

Working Out at Home Instead of a Fitness Center!

Most women I talk to say they have several pieces of home exercise equipment. Most of it is in their basement, garage or closet gathering dust. A sales representative from a huge home equipment company told me, "research has found that the average life use of a piece of home exercise equipment is only five hours of actual use".

That means the most people do not use home equipment. Exercise equipment is only a tool and you need to keep changing your routine to keep your exercise program interesting. Exercising at home is seldom effective because of the interruptions from the telephone, family and a thousand other things. You will have better results in the right type of fitness center. Do not forget the social aspects. In a survey hundreds of committed exercisers were questions about why they keep exercising. Eighty five percent said "social reasons kept them coming". For this reason always try to get your close friends involved with you.

Want a personal trainer? Not all personal trainers are equal. Most give their clients the same type of workout they would do. Most are young and like most young people they consider themselves indestructible. Many have very little experience dealing with the overweight or de-conditioned market. They would be a great drill instructor at a marine boot camp or football training camp. Dealing with overweight women's problems, no way. You need some one with experience dealing with the overweight. It is totally different than the athlete.

Toning Tables

These are assisted motorized exercise machines. The story goes that these exercise machines were invented years ago by a doctor for his crippled daughter. He wanted to help prevent additional atrophy to her muscles. Then discovered these machines helped other people.

They noticed that some of the overweight ladies started to gain strength while losing inches. More and more overweight and older women started using them on their exercise routine. The principles is you gently push against the machine as it moves toward you and you can do hundreds of enjoyable repetitions . Women really enjoy using these machines.

How it works, the motor is more powerful than you or I am, by pushing against it as it moves, you control the resistance. For example most all seriously overweight women are unable to do sit ups. The toning tables are easy and supportive.

Why Is Pride Important?

Which woman is going to feel better about herself? The one that exercises faithfully, maintains her ideal weight and looks good, or the woman who goes on diet after diet, gives up and develops a learned helplessness? A woman who loses the battle much too often will devour all the food insight to drown her sorrows?

Self-esteem comes from achieving difficult things. Naturally the woman who achieves a level of physical fitness feels better about herself. The woman who gives up on herself probably feels a certain amount of emotional pain.

Resolve that is exercised becomes stronger. Resolve that is abandoned become weaker and weaker.

Concentrating on changing you mindset is far easier than trying to give up food you want to eat.

To win the game of getting to your best physical condition and achieving your ideal weight, you have to understand why you want to do it in the first place. There is only one person who can provide you with the power to do this, and that person is you.

No one can win this battle for you, but you! I can help teach you how to fight, but "you must do it".

When you wake up in the morning, start exercising and think of all the reasons you are grateful. Visualize and think of all the people who are important to you in your life and all the things you have to feel grateful for. The more you do this, the easier it becomes.

You will feel the negative feelings melting away and the stress will start leaving your body. Think of why you like your body and why you cherish yourself. Mentally, experience the good times of your life. Think about when you were in better shape and more active.

If negative thoughts come up, question "What can I learn from this, and how can I use it to make my life better?" Remember, the quality of your life is equal to the quality of the questions you ask yourself.

Visualize the cherished moments of your life. In your mind's eye visualize the light very bright. It will make the mental background emotionally intense and strong.

One of the keys to fighting and winning the battle is to be prepared, then pace yourself. Do not try to change years into days; you can't. You will only burn yourself out.

Doing the "oxygen stimulator" reduces stress. You feel better about yourself because you are more positive. I have had women tell me that they find themselves treating their families better. Even people come up to them and say, how much more fun they are to be around and that they notice a big improvement.

When you start to care for and cherish yourself more, then you have more love to give to cherish others. It is a wonderful cycle that keeps coming back to you.

Keep doing this and never give up. The better you feel, the better you want to feel. Do not take it for granted. If you do you will stop reaffirming your gratitude. Then the negative forces little by little will direct your mind. The news and the television commercials on food will suck your resolve from you. Then everything will be lost, except the thirty, forty or fifty additional pounds will have gain.

The question is not if your extra weight will damage your body, but when? Almost all obese women suffer after reaching fifty or sixty years of age. The damage is often so severe nothing can be done for them.

They have injured their bodies so badly they can hardly move. Physically they are a disaster. At that point it is too late.

It is not too late for you if you realize lifestyle changes with mindset and with different priorities. If you do not constantly reaffirm your goals and priorities, then others will do it for you.

The average thirty-five year old woman has seen two thousand accumulated hours of food commercials on television. Using emotional leverage, their objective is to get you to be a trained "consumer garbage disposal" for their garbage. The more you eat, the more money junk food advertisers make.

What would happen if you had seen over two thousand hours of psychological stimulating reasons to exercise and be healthier?

Would you be different? Of course you would be! You would look incredible, feel energetic, and be a happy, positive, vivacious individual.

Health clubs do not have the kind of money to do a lot of advertising. People must eat to stay alive, but they need less food and more exercise. If you want productive thoughts in your mind, you must consciously put them there. No one else has the power or ability to help you, but you.

Like any good fighter, you must psychologically refuse to be beaten. Take pride in your potential as a human being. You can achieve anything you set your mind to. You must do this for you. Refuse to see yourself as a victim, and then you are able to win. Just as in fighting, you have to know your own limitations and be realistic. Try to get better not perfect. Set yourself up to win. The way to do this is to enjoy the process. Let it be your reward. Those who do not love the process give up. Those who give up do not succeed. If you fail, try again. Losing weight will always be a fight for most of us. Yet, we are worth it.

In the past ten to twenty years the number of obese people has increased tremendously. The forces to overeat are strong, so strong that ninety five percent of those who lose weight gain it all back within one or two years. We have never been taught how to manage our impulses. We need to manage ourselves if we are to be healthy, trim, and physically fit.

I fought the weight battle. I have also heard many horror stories from overweight women. But what disturbs me most is the increase in obesity in children. It breaks my heart to see small children suffer because the quality of their life is compromised by a serious weight problem.

As a child I was lucky. We did not have a television set in our home until I was around thirteen. There was only one channel that came on in the evening. Our time was occupied in sports, play, and running in the woods. Obesity in kids was rare. We were busy and having too much fun to be concerned about food.

Now some parents use their television sets as babysitters. Between the television and the computer, people are not nearly as active.

What compounds the problem is the advertising of food directed to the children. As I said earlier the problem is so bad that in one Scandinavian country. I read it is illegal to direct television advertising toward children.

Just think, the average television program is between one quarter and one-third advertising. Half of that is food advertising using every psychological hook they can to emotionally get people to eat so that they can make more money.

We have made it illegal to direct television advertising from tobacco companies to children. Drugs are illegal and alcohol is illegal to sell to children.

Many children view television food commercials for over an hour a day. For junk food advertisers to use misleading and dangerous psychological tactics can be physically and/or psychologically damaging to our children, which is wrong.

I think it is worth repeating that on the Internet I found statistics that the total budget for all fruits and vegetable food advertising in the United States in 1996 was less than one million dollars. While McDonalds alone spent over five hundred and fifty million dollars on advertising in 1996.

Often, if you see an obese child you see an obese parent. It is not only genetics the parent passes on to the child but bad habits. If the parents want to eat themselves into a living hell that is their business. They have no right to harm their child and to teach them bad habits that eventually become difficult to break. If you care about your child then care enough to set the very best example that you can. Love your children enough not to constantly stuff them full of junk food.

Recently I have written letters to senators, congressmen, and governors urging the research of causes of obesity.

Obesity is having a damaging effect on Americans' quality of life. We just understand all the reasons so that we can have a better chance of successfully fighting back. Food advertisements are not the sole problem, but they can contribute to us eating ten percent more calories. These calories can add up and will most likely turn into fat. Over a period of years they will add up to a substantial amount of pounds.

One thing is for certain, the problem of obesity in our children is far worse than the general public understands. We should care for and protect our children, even if we do neglect ourselves. How can we help our children if we are not good role models?

Think about it, appreciate yourself, and appreciate your children. Take care of all of you. Stop being a "patsy to food." Stop eating junk food as a means to reduce stress or to distract you from life's problems. Food is not love, it is fuel for your body. Get off the path of self-destruction because too much food is nothing more but a slow poison.

In USA Today, January 28, 2001, there was a short article, "Diabetes, Obesity Near Epidemic Levels." I tell everyone that I care. I question if they care. Do You? Then I tell them lets do something about it.

This reminds me of two experiences that are seared into my memory. One of our members while riding the exercise bicycle was having her young daughter sitting on the floor next to her. This was clearly against the club rules. They needed to be in the children's play area.

I went over to her and told her it was very dangerous for her daughter to be there. She said "It is just fine for my daughter to be here. She does not like the kids play area and she cries every time I put her in there. I spent several minutes trying to convince the mother to take her daughter to the safer children's play area. I finally gave up being no match for the mother persistence. I was not in a mood to argue with her any longer.

As I started back to my desk, I heard a blood curdling scream. The young daughter had poked her finger into the sprocket of the exercise bike and it was cut off.

The child was screaming and the mother started crying, repeating over and over to her daughter how sorry she was. She said the same thing to me as she left for the hospital. That was forty years ago. I feel almost certain that every time the mother sees that hand with the missing finger she feels guilty. Knowing the finger would still be there if she had chosen to listen, not argue. What can happen eventually will. By her dismissing danger, did not make it go away. She took the path of the least resistance with her daughter and they both suffered because of it.

The next memory was about when I operated clubs for both men and women. One lady member brought in her husband. She wanted me to convince her husband that he should join because he need to take better care of himself and to get more exercise.

I had no luck with him. He insisted that he got all the exercise he needed, but he said he was glad that his wife was working out.

About six weeks later I saw his wife when she came in to exercise. I asked about her husband, but she broke down crying. She said that he had died of a heart attack three weeks ago. Sobbing she said "He was only 41 years old," She got to me when she said "I wonder if he would still be alive today I you had been able to persuade him to exercise? He needed it so badly," she went on saying.

Those words still haunt me, I have no way of knowing if he had started to exercise if it would have save his life, or not. But one thing is certain, no matter how badly I want to help you, you must do it yourself.

Exercise And
Weight Loss Program

Works only for as long as you work them.

POWER PRINCIPLES YOU CAN USE.

1. Six times a day do the "oxygen stimulator" as I previously described.

2. When working out, visually and mentally affirm what you have to be grateful for. Think of ways to improve your life. Celebrate your body. Think of the little things one after another. The more you appreciate yourself, the more you are apt to take care of yourself.

3. Overweight people don't stay fat when they work for fitness centers. The only fat people I know of in our business are family members who do not care enough to practice what they preach.

4. If you believe in fitness and being in shape, the best way you can motivate yourself is to start regularly motivating others.

5. If you usually see thirty minutes a day of food commercials on television and you have a weight problem, then start spending thirty

minutes a day trying to motivate as many people as possible to get and to stay in shape. This will strengthen your reasons by you selling yourself on the idea of getting and keeping fit. Who knows! You might want to work full or part time with us.

Each night listen to guided imagery cassette tapes or self-hypnosis audiocassettes, and listen to their strategies to help reach your ideal weight and level of fitness.

"A combination of things works better than just one thing."

To insure success all four of these tools must be used.

One reason most people who are motivated to start a weight loss program usually fail, is they just assume that their motivation will continue. As I said earlier it is like the sun. It shines bright, then disappears, then reappears, and then disappears. This causes weight to do the same.

The desire must shine from the inside. Your will, your mindset, and your desires, reside there. Focus on them, pump them up several times a day and your success will astonish you!

My web site.www.lifeislikeaturtle.com
My email address fitness@swcp.com

God Bless, and now become the type of person you deserve to be. **"Happy, Trim, and Fit for Life."**

In Review

Nowhere in the human body is there a strong biological urge or trigger to exercise for physical fitness. In fact, the impulse is to conserve energy.

AGREE_____DISAGREE_____

(As compared to the drive food or sex, because adequate physical activity was always a requirement just to survive for our ancestors.)

Food advertisers spend billions of dollars on advertising to condition us to turn to food and to associate food with pleasure so we will eat more and they will make a large profit.

AGREE_____DISAGREE_____

Since there is no human impulse or drive to exercise regularly, unless we deliberately reinforce those reasons, we should exercise and associate pleasure to those reasons on a regular basis. We most likely will give up our exercise and fitness efforts and not look or feel our best, if we don't.

AGREE_____DISAGREE_____

People don't overeat because they are hungry, but because they are stressed or faced with boredom. The more overweight they become the more stressed and unhappy people get, again turning to food for comfort.

AGREE_____DISAGREE_____

If a person currently has a weight problem, they must lose that weight or eventually
suffer from the affects of obesity.

AGREE_____DISAGREE_____

Even though decisions don't have calories. The calories in food can't hurt you unless you decide to put it in your mouth.

AGREE_____DISAGREE_____

If I don't consciously and effectively motivate myself each day to exercise and to keep my weight under control, it will not happen.

AGREE_____DISAGREE_____

The better I feel about myself, the more likely I am to take care of myself.

AGREE_____DISAGREE_____

The reason that traditional weight loss efforts have a 95% failure ratio is because they focus on the wrong thing and take the wrong approach.

AGREE_____DISAGREE_____

The quality of your life is equal to the quality of the questions you ask yourself

Shocked Into Action

12 quality questions about
what I want to think about.

I want to stay fat   Yes_____ No_____

I need to lose__pounds   Yes_____ No_____

I want to die from
my weight problem?   Yes_____ No_____

 Do I care about how I look?   Yes_____ No_____

I want to suffer pain from
a future knee problem.   Yes_____ No_____

I want future back pain caused from being
severely overweight   Yes_____ No_____

I want to develop diabetes as a result of my
weight problem   Yes_____ No_____

Would Members of my family be proud
of me if I personally took control of my
weight problem.   Yes_____ No_____

Do my loved ones blame and
resent me for not conquering my
weight problem?   Yes_____ No_____

Does being overweight hurt my appearance?
My health? My self respect?   Yes_____ No_____

As a human being, do I consider
myself worth the effort?   Yes_____ No_____

When I die or become seriously handicapped
from being overweight, will this put a needless
hardship on my loved ones and will they be angry
with me because I did this?   Yes_____ No_____

95% of people who lose weight
gain it all back within 2 years, plus more

What has to happen to get and
keep that weight off?

1. Reduce Stress- 43% of the women reduce stress by eating.

2. Feel good about yourself and be happy. Improve self-esteem.

3. Get excited about your future–depressed people turn to food for comfort.

4. Eliminate the power of food advertisers over you. Replace destructive television and radio junk food commercials with positive health and fitness messages.

5. Be pro active constantly. Sell yourself on fitness and get excited about your life. Encourage others to do the same, this will reinforce you.

THIS IS YOR LADDER, STEP BY STEP. YOU CAN MAKE THE IMPOSSIBLE, POSSIBLE!

My Secret Wish List

Make a list of 7 people who are important to you, those individuals that you want to be a positive influence on their health, fitness, and life goals over the next 12 months.

You will lead and inspire people by your words and examples. Out of 7, your ultimate goal is to have a major impact on at least three of their lives.

Remember, if you don't talk about your health, fitness or personal achievement, you will not think about it.

Put your credibility on the line, so you can't fail; refuse to give up. This way you will walk your talk.

Name_____Why I am committed to helping them?

_____

_____

_____

Name_____Why I am
committed to helping them?

_____

_____

_____

Name_____Why I am
committed to helping them?

_____

_____

_____

Name_____Why I am
committed to helping them?

_____

_____

_____

Name_____Why I am
committed to helping them?

_____

_____

_____

Name_____Why I am
committed to helping them?

_____

_____

_____

Name_____Why   I   am
committed to helping them?

_____

_____

_____

I hereby promise this to myself.

Signed_____Date:_____

List Time and Dates

You Listened To
"Make It Happen: Tapes"

Tape #   Date: Tape   # Date:

_____   _____

_____   _____

_____   _____

_____   _____

_____   _____

_____   _____

_____   _____

_____   _____

_____   _____

_____   _____

_____   _____

_____   _____

_____   _____

_____   _____

_____   _____

_____   _____

_____   _____

_____   _____

_____   _____

List Time and Dates

You Listened To
"Make It Happen: Tapes"

Tape #	Date:	Tape	# Date:

List Time and Dates

You Listened To
"Make It Happen: Tapes"

Tape #	Date:	Tape	# Date:
_____	_____	_____	_____
_____	_____	_____	_____
_____	_____	_____	_____
_____	_____	_____	_____
_____	_____	_____	_____
_____	_____	_____	_____
_____	_____	_____	_____
_____	_____	_____	_____
_____	_____	_____	_____
_____	_____	_____	_____
_____	_____	_____	_____
_____	_____	_____	_____
_____	_____	_____	_____
_____	_____	_____	_____
_____	_____	_____	_____
_____	_____	_____	_____
_____	_____	_____	_____
_____	_____	_____	_____
_____	_____	_____	_____

List Time and Dates

You Listened To
"Make It Happen: Tapes"

Tape #	Date:	Tape	# Date:
_____	_____	_____	_____
_____	_____	_____	_____
_____	_____	_____	_____
_____	_____	_____	_____
_____	_____	_____	_____
_____	_____	_____	_____
_____	_____	_____	_____
_____	_____	_____	_____
_____	_____	_____	_____
_____	_____	_____	_____
_____	_____	_____	_____
_____	_____	_____	_____
_____	_____	_____	_____
_____	_____	_____	_____
_____	_____	_____	_____
_____	_____	_____	_____
_____	_____	_____	_____
_____	_____	_____	_____
_____	_____	_____	_____
_____	_____	_____	_____
_____	_____	_____	_____

List Time and Dates

You Listened To
"Make It Happen: Tapes"

Tape #   Date: Tape   # Date:

——————————   ——————————
——————————   ——————————
——————————   ——————————
——————————   ——————————
——————————   ——————————
——————————   ——————————
——————————   ——————————
——————————   ——————————
——————————   ——————————
——————————   ——————————
——————————   ——————————
——————————   ——————————
——————————   ——————————
——————————   ——————————
——————————   ——————————
——————————   ——————————
——————————   ——————————
——————————   ——————————
——————————   ——————————

List Time and Dates

You Listened To
"Make It Happen: Tapes"

Tape #   Date: Tape   # Date:

_____ _____

_____ _____

_____ _____

_____ _____

_____ _____

_____ _____

_____ _____

_____ _____

_____ _____

_____ _____

_____ _____

_____ _____

_____ _____

_____ _____

_____ _____

_____ _____

_____ _____

_____ _____

_____ _____

List Time and Dates

You Listened To
"Make It Happen: Tapes"

Tape #	Date:	Tape	# Date:

List Time and Dates

You Listened To
"Make It Happen: Tapes"

Tape #	Date:	Tape	# Date:

List Time and Dates

You Listened To
"Make It Happen: Tapes"

Tape #	Date:	Tape	# Date:

List Time and Dates

You Listened To
"Make It Happen: Tapes"

Tape #	Date:	Tape	# Date:

Negative Thoughts Diary

What was the thought?

_____

_____

_____

What triggered the thought (what happened right before the thought?

_____

_____

_____

How did the thought make me feel?

_____

_____

_____

What did I do next (what action or behavior)?

_____

_____

_____

How did I see myself during this time?

_____

_____

_____

Negative Thoughts Diary

What was the thought?

_____

_____

_____

What triggered the thought (what happened right before the thought?

_____

_____

_____

How did the thought make me feel?

_____

_____

_____

What did I do next (what action or behavior)?

_____

_____

_____

How did I see myself during this time?

_____

_____

_____

Negative Thoughts Diary

What was the thought?

_____

_____

_____

What triggered the thought (what happened right before the thought?

_____

_____

_____

How did the thought make me feel?

_____

_____

_____

What did I do next (what action or behavior)?

_____

_____

_____

How did I see myself during this time?

_____

_____

_____

Negative Thoughts Diary

What was the thought?

_____

_____

_____

What triggered the thought (what happened right before the thought?

_____

_____

_____

How did the thought make me feel?

_____

_____

_____

What did I do next (what action or behavior)?

_____

_____

_____

How did I see myself during this time?

_____

_____

_____

Negative Thoughts Diary

What was the thought?

_____

_____

_____

What triggered the thought (what happened right before the thought?

_____

_____

_____

How did the thought make me feel?

_____

_____

_____

What did I do next (what action or behavior)?

_____

_____

_____

How did I see myself during this time?

_____

_____

_____

_____

Negative Thoughts Diary

What was the thought?

_____

_____

_____

What triggered the thought (what happened right before the thought?

_____

_____

_____

How did the thought make me feel?

_____

_____

_____

What did I do next (what action or behavior)?

_____

_____

_____

How did I see myself during this time?

_____

_____

_____

Negative Thoughts Diary

What was the thought?

_____

_____

_____

What triggered the thought (what happened right before the thought?

_____

_____

_____

How did the thought make me feel?

_____

_____

_____

What did I do next (what action or behavior)?

_____

_____

_____

How did I see myself during this time?

_____

_____

_____

Negative Thoughts Diary

What was the thought?

_____

_____

_____

What triggered the thought (what happened right before the thought?

_____

_____

_____

How did the thought make me feel?

_____

_____

_____

What did I do next (what action or behavior)?

_____

_____

_____

How did I see myself during this time?

_____

_____

_____

Negative Thoughts Diary

What was the thought?

_____

_____

_____

What triggered the thought (what happened right before the thought?

_____

_____

_____

How did the thought make me feel?

_____

_____

_____

What did I do next (what action or behavior)?

_____

_____

_____

How did I see myself during this time?

_____

_____

_____

Negative Thoughts Diary

What was the thought?

_____

_____

_____

What triggered the thought (what happened right before the thought?

_____

_____

_____

How did the thought make me feel?

_____

_____

_____

What did I do next (what action or behavior)?

_____

_____

_____

How did I see myself during this time?

_____

_____

_____

Weekly Food Diary

FROM _____ TO _____

	Breakfast	Lunch	Dinner	Snacks	Water
Sunday					
Monday					
Tuesday					
Wednesday					
Thursday					
Friday					
Saturday					

Weekly Food Diary

FROM _____ TO _____

	Breakfast	Lunch	Dinner	Snacks	Water
Sunday					
Monday					
Tuesday					
Wednesday					
Thursday					
Friday					
Saturday					

Weekly Food Diary

FROM _____ TO _____

	Breakfast	Lunch	Dinner	Snacks	Water
Sunday					
Monday					
Tuesday					
Wednesday					
Thursday					
Friday					
Saturday					

Weekly Food Diary

FROM _____ TO _____

	Breakfast	Lunch	Dinner	Snacks	Water
Sunday					
Monday					
Tuesday					
Wednesday					
Thursday					
Friday					
Saturday					

Weekly Food Diary

FROM _____ TO _____

	Breakfast	Lunch	Dinner	Snacks	Water
Sunday					
Monday					
Tuesday					
Wednesday					
Thursday					
Friday					
Saturday					

Weekly Food Diary

FROM _____ TO _____

	Breakfast	Lunch	Dinner	Snacks	Water
Sunday					
Monday					
Tuesday					
Wednesday					
Thursday					
Friday					
Saturday					

Weekly Food Diary

FROM _____ TO _____

	Breakfast	Lunch	Dinner	Snacks	Water
Sunday					
Monday					
Tuesday					
Wednesday					
Thursday					
Friday					
Saturday					

Weekly Food Diary

FROM _____ TO _____

	Breakfast	Lunch	Dinner	Snacks	Water
Sunday					
Monday					
Tuesday					
Wednesday					
Thursday					
Friday					
Saturday					

Weekly Food Diary

FROM _____ TO _____

	Breakfast	Lunch	Dinner	Snacks	Water
Sunday					
Monday					
Tuesday					
Wednesday					
Thursday					
Friday					
Saturday					

Weekly Food Diary

FROM _____ TO _____

	Breakfast	Lunch	Dinner	Snacks	Water
Sunday					
Monday					
Tuesday					
Wednesday					
Thursday					
Friday					
Saturday					

Weekly Food Diary

FROM _____ TO _____

	Breakfast	Lunch	Dinner	Snacks	Water
Sunday					
Monday					
Tuesday					
Wednesday					
Thursday					
Friday					
Saturday					

Weekly Food Diary

FROM _____ TO _____

	Breakfast	Lunch	Dinner	Snacks	Water
Sunday					
Monday					
Tuesday					
Wednesday					
Thursday					
Friday					
Saturday					

Weekly Food Diary

FROM _____ TO _____

	Breakfast	Lunch	Dinner	Snacks	Water
Sunday					
Monday					
Tuesday					
Wednesday					
Thursday					
Friday					
Saturday					

Weekly Food Diary

FROM _____ TO _____

	Breakfast	Lunch	Dinner	Snacks	Water
Sunday					
Monday					
Tuesday					
Wednesday					
Thursday					
Friday					
Saturday					

Oxygen Stimulator 1st____2nd____3rd____4th____5th____6th____

Keeping focused...If you don't talk about it, you won't think about fitness. Build a new support group and a new attitude.
Keep selling yourself on fitness and health by talking about how much you enjoy exercising and its benefits. Do this for at least 6 times a day for 90 days. Enough time to develop new habits and attitudes and beliefs. If you don't, then there is up to a 95% chance of failure. If you fail to follow through, just keep trying.

Daily Log

Date_____   _____

1st-Time	Talked to:
2nd Time	Talked to:
3rd Time	Talked to:
4th Time	Talked to:
5th Time	Talked to:
6th Time	Talked to:
7th Time	Talked to:
8th Time	Talked to:
9th Time	Talked to:
10th Time	Talked to:
11th Time	Talked to:

Oxygen Stimulator 1st____2nd____3rd____4th____5th____6th____

Keeping focused…If you don't talk about it, you won't think about fitness. Build a new support group and a new attitude.
Keep selling yourself on fitness and health by talking about how much you enjoy exercising and its benefits. Do this for at least 6 times a day for 90 days. Enough time to develop new habits and attitudes and beliefs. If you don't, then there is up to a 95% chance of failure. If you fail to follow through, just keep trying.

Daily Log

Date_____   _____

1st-Time   Talked to: _____

2nd Time _____   Talked to: _____

3rd Time _____   Talked to: _____

4th Time _____   Talked to: _____

5th Time _____   Talked to: _____

6th Time _____   Talked to: _____

7th Time _____   Talked to: _____

8th Time _____   Talked to: _____

9th Time _____   Talked to: _____

10th Time _____   Talked to: _____

11th Time _____   Talked to: _____

Oxygen Stimulator 1st____2nd____3rd____4th____5th____6th____

Keeping focused…If you don't talk about it, you won't think about fitness. Build a new support group and a new attitude.

Keep selling yourself on fitness and health by talking about how much you enjoy exercising and its benefits. Do this for at least 6 times a day for 90 days. Enough time to develop new habits and attitudes and beliefs. If you don't, then there is up to a 95% chance of failure. If you fail to follow through, just keep trying.

Daily Log

Date_____   _____

1st-Time	Talked to:
2nd Time	Talked to:
3rd Time	Talked to:
4th Time	Talked to:
5th Time	Talked to:
6th Time	Talked to:
7th Time	Talked to:
8th Time	Talked to:
9th Time	Talked to:
10th Time	Talked to:
11th Time	Talked to:

Oxygen Stimulator 1st_____2nd_____3rd_____4th_____5th_____6th_____

Keeping focused…If you don't talk about it, you won't think about fitness. Build a new support group and a new attitude.

Keep selling yourself on fitness and health by talking about how much you enjoy exercising and its benefits. Do this for at least 6 times a day for 90 days. Enough time to develop new habits and attitudes and beliefs. If you don't, then there is up to a 95% chance of failure. If you fail to follow through, just keep trying.

Daily Log

Date_____   _____

1st-Time	Talked to:
2nd Time	Talked to:
3rd Time	Talked to:
4th Time	Talked to:
5th Time	Talked to:
6th Time	Talked to:
7th Time	Talked to:
8th Time	Talked to:
9th Time	Talked to:
10th Time	Talked to:
11th Time	Talked to:

Oxygen Stimulator 1st____2nd____3rd____4th____5th____6th____

Keeping focused…If you don't talk about it, you won't think about fitness. Build a new support group and a new attitude.

Keep selling yourself on fitness and health by talking about how much you enjoy exercising and its benefits. Do this for at least 6 times a day for 90 days. Enough time to develop new habits and attitudes and beliefs. If you don't, then there is up to a 95% chance of failure. If you fail to follow through, just keep trying.

Daily Log

Date_____   _____

1st-Time	Talked to:
2nd Time	Talked to:
3rd Time	Talked to:
4th Time	Talked to:
5th Time	Talked to:
6th Time	Talked to:
7th Time	Talked to:
8th Time	Talked to:
9th Time	Talked to:
10th Time	Talked to:
11th Time	Talked to:

Oxygen Stimulator 1st_____2nd_____3rd_____4th_____5th_____6th_____

Keeping focused…If you don't talk about it, you won't think about fitness. Build a new support group and a new attitude.

Keep selling yourself on fitness and health by talking about how much you enjoy exercising and its benefits. Do this for at least 6 times a day for 90 days. Enough time to develop new habits and attitudes and beliefs. If you don't, then there is up to a 95% chance of failure. If you fail to follow through, just keep trying.

Daily Log

Date_____   _____

1st-Time	Talked to:
2nd Time	Talked to:
3rd Time	Talked to:
4th Time	Talked to:
5th Time	Talked to:
6th Time	Talked to:
7th Time	Talked to:
8th Time	Talked to:
9th Time	Talked to:
10th Time	Talked to:
11th Time	Talked to:

Oxygen Stimulator 1st____2nd____3rd____4th____5th____6th____

Keeping focused…If you don't talk about it, you won't think about fitness. Build a new support group and a new attitude.

Keep selling yourself on fitness and health by talking about how much you enjoy exercising and its benefits. Do this for at least 6 times a day for 90 days. Enough time to develop new habits and attitudes and beliefs. If you don't, then there is up to a 95% chance of failure. If you fail to follow through, just keep trying.

Daily Log

Date_____   _____

1st-Time   Talked to: _____

2nd Time   Talked to: _____

3rd Time   Talked to: _____

4th Time   Talked to: _____

5th Time   Talked to: _____

6th Time   Talked to: _____

7th Time   Talked to: _____

8th Time   Talked to: _____

9th Time   Talked to: _____

10th Time   Talked to: _____

11th Time   Talked to: _____

Oxygen Stimulator 1st_____2nd_____3rd_____4th_____5th_____6th_____

Keeping focused…If you don't talk about it, you won't think about fitness. Build a new support group and a new attitude.

Keep selling yourself on fitness and health by talking about how much you enjoy exercising and its benefits. Do this for at least 6 times a day for 90 days. Enough time to develop new habits and attitudes and beliefs. If you don't, then there is up to a 95% chance of failure. If you fail to follow through, just keep trying.

Daily Log

Date_____   _____

1st-Time	Talked to:
2nd Time	Talked to:
3rd Time	Talked to:
4th Time	Talked to:
5th Time	Talked to:
6th Time	Talked to:
7th Time	Talked to:
8th Time	Talked to:
9th Time	Talked to:
10th Time	Talked to:
11th Time	Talked to:

Oxygen Stimulator 1st_____2nd_____3rd_____4th_____5th_____6th_____

Keeping focused…If you don't talk about it, you won't think about fitness. Build a new support group and a new attitude.

Keep selling yourself on fitness and health by talking about how much you enjoy exercising and its benefits. Do this for at least 6 times a day for 90 days. Enough time to develop new habits and attitudes and beliefs. If you don't, then there is up to a 95% chance of failure. If you fail to follow through, just keep trying.

Daily Log

Date_____   _____

1st-Time	Talked to:
2nd Time	Talked to:
3rd Time	Talked to:
4th Time	Talked to:
5th Time	Talked to:
6th Time	Talked to:
7th Time	Talked to:
8th Time	Talked to:
9th Time	Talked to:
10th Time	Talked to:
11th Time	Talked to:

Oxygen Stimulator 1st____2nd____3rd____4th____5th____6th____

Keeping focused…If you don't talk about it, you won't think about fitness. Build a new support group and a new attitude.

Keep selling yourself on fitness and health by talking about how much you enjoy exercising and its benefits. Do this for at least 6 times a day for 90 days. Enough time to develop new habits and attitudes and beliefs. If you don't, then there is up to a 95% chance of failure. If you fail to follow through, just keep trying.

Daily Log

Date_____   _____

1st-Time	Talked to:
2nd Time	Talked to:
3rd Time	Talked to:
4th Time	Talked to:
5th Time	Talked to:
6th Time	Talked to:
7th Time	Talked to:
8th Time	Talked to:
9th Time	Talked to:
10th Time	Talked to:
11th Time	Talked to:

Oxygen Stimulator 1st____2nd____3rd____4th____5th____6th____

Keeping focused…If you don't talk about it, you won't think about fitness. Build a new support group and a new attitude.
Keep selling yourself on fitness and health by talking about how much you enjoy exercising and its benefits. Do this for at least 6 times a day for 90 days. Enough time to develop new habits and attitudes and beliefs. If you don't, then there is up to a 95% chance of failure. If you fail to follow through, just keep trying.

Daily Log

Date_____   _____

1st-Time	Talked to:
2nd Time	Talked to:
3rd Time	Talked to:
4th Time	Talked to:
5th Time	Talked to:
6th Time	Talked to:
7th Time	Talked to:
8th Time	Talked to:
9th Time	Talked to:
10th Time	Talked to:
11th Time	Talked to:

Oxygen Stimulator 1st____2nd____3rd____4th____5th____6th____

Keeping focused…If you don't talk about it, you won't think about fitness. Build a new support group and a new attitude.

Keep selling yourself on fitness and health by talking about how much you enjoy exercising and its benefits. Do this for at least 6 times a day for 90 days. Enough time to develop new habits and attitudes and beliefs. If you don't, then there is up to a 95% chance of failure. If you fail to follow through, just keep trying.

Daily Log

Date_____   _____

1st-Time	Talked to:
2nd Time	Talked to:
3rd Time	Talked to:
4th Time	Talked to:
5th Time	Talked to:
6th Time	Talked to:
7th Time	Talked to:
8th Time	Talked to:
9th Time	Talked to:
10th Time	Talked to:
11th Time	Talked to:

Oxygen Stimulator 1st____2nd____3rd____4th____5th____6th____

Keeping focused…If you don't talk about it, you won't think about fitness. Build a new support group and a new attitude.

Keep selling yourself on fitness and health by talking about how much you enjoy exercising and its benefits. Do this for at least 6 times a day for 90 days. Enough time to develop new habits and attitudes and beliefs. If you don't, then there is up to a 95% chance of failure. If you fail to follow through, just keep trying.

Daily Log

Date_____   _____

1st-Time	Talked to:
2nd Time	Talked to:
3rd Time	Talked to:
4th Time	Talked to:
5th Time	Talked to:
6th Time	Talked to:
7th Time	Talked to:
8th Time	Talked to:
9th Time	Talked to:
10th Time	Talked to:
11th Time	Talked to:

Oxygen Stimulator 1st____2nd____3rd____4th____5th____6th____

Keeping focused…If you don't talk about it, you won't think about fitness. Build a new support group and a new attitude.

Keep selling yourself on fitness and health by talking about how much you enjoy exercising and its benefits. Do this for at least 6 times a day for 90 days. Enough time to develop new habits and attitudes and beliefs. If you don't, then there is up to a 95% chance of failure. If you fail to follow through, just keep trying.

Daily Log

Date_____   _____

1st-Time	Talked to:
2nd Time	Talked to:
3rd Time	Talked to:
4th Time	Talked to:
5th Time	Talked to:
6th Time	Talked to:
7th Time	Talked to:
8th Time	Talked to:
9th Time	Talked to:
10th Time	Talked to:
11th Time	Talked to:

Oxygen Stimulator 1st_____2nd_____3rd_____4th_____5th_____6th_____

Keeping focused…If you don't talk about it, you won't think about fitness. Build a new support group and a new attitude.

Keep selling yourself on fitness and health by talking about how much you enjoy exercising and its benefits. Do this for at least 6 times a day for 90 days. Enough time to develop new habits and attitudes and beliefs. If you don't, then there is up to a 95% chance of failure. If you fail to follow through, just keep trying.

Daily Log

Date_____   _____

1st-Time	Talked to:
2nd Time	Talked to:
3rd Time	Talked to:
4th Time	Talked to:
5th Time	Talked to:
6th Time	Talked to:
7th Time	Talked to:
8th Time	Talked to:
9th Time	Talked to:
10th Time	Talked to:
11th Time	Talked to:

Oxygen Stimulator 1st____2nd____3rd____4th____5th____6th____

Keeping focused…If you don't talk about it, you won't think about fitness. Build a new support group and a new attitude.

Keep selling yourself on fitness and health by talking about how much you enjoy exercising and its benefits. Do this for at least 6 times a day for 90 days. Enough time to develop new habits and attitudes and beliefs. If you don't, then there is up to a 95% chance of failure. If you fail to follow through, just keep trying.

Daily Log

Date_____   _____

1st-Time	Talked to:
2nd Time	Talked to:
3rd Time	Talked to:
4th Time	Talked to:
5th Time	Talked to:
6th Time	Talked to:
7th Time	Talked to:
8th Time	Talked to:
9th Time	Talked to:
10th Time	Talked to:
11th Time	Talked to:

Oxygen Stimulator 1st_____2nd_____3rd_____4th_____5th_____6th_____

Keeping focused…If you don't talk about it, you won't think about fitness. Build a new support group and a new attitude.

Keep selling yourself on fitness and health by talking about how much you enjoy exercising and its benefits. Do this for at least 6 times a day for 90 days. Enough time to develop new habits and attitudes and beliefs. If you don't, then there is up to a 95% chance of failure. If you fail to follow through, just keep trying.

Daily Log

Date_____   _____

1st-Time	Talked to:
2nd Time	Talked to:
3rd Time	Talked to:
4th Time	Talked to:
5th Time	Talked to:
6th Time	Talked to:
7th Time	Talked to:
8th Time	Talked to:
9th Time	Talked to:
10th Time	Talked to:
11th Time	Talked to:

Oxygen Stimulator 1st____2nd____3rd____4th____5th____6th____

Keeping focused…If you don't talk about it, you won't think about fitness. Build a new support group and a new attitude.

Keep selling yourself on fitness and health by talking about how much you enjoy exercising and its benefits. Do this for at least 6 times a day for 90 days. Enough time to develop new habits and attitudes and beliefs. If you don't, then there is up to a 95% chance of failure. If you fail to follow through, just keep trying.

Daily Log

Date_____   _____

1st-Time	Talked to:
2nd Time	Talked to:
3rd Time	Talked to:
4th Time	Talked to:
5th Time	Talked to:
6th Time	Talked to:
7th Time	Talked to:
8th Time	Talked to:
9th Time	Talked to:
10th Time	Talked to:
11th Time	Talked to:

Oxygen Stimulator 1st_____2nd_____3rd_____4th_____5th_____6th_____

Keeping focused…If you don't talk about it, you won't think about fitness. Build a new support group and a new attitude.

Keep selling yourself on fitness and health by talking about how much you enjoy exercising and its benefits. Do this for at least 6 times a day for 90 days. Enough time to develop new habits and attitudes and beliefs. If you don't, then there is up to a 95% chance of failure. If you fail to follow through, just keep trying.

Daily Log

Date_____   _____

1st-Time	Talked to:
2nd Time	Talked to:
3rd Time	Talked to:
4th Time	Talked to:
5th Time	Talked to:
6th Time	Talked to:
7th Time	Talked to:
8th Time	Talked to:
9th Time	Talked to:
10th Time	Talked to:
11th Time	Talked to:

Oxygen Stimulator 1st____2nd____3rd____4th____5th____6th____

Keeping focused…If you don't talk about it, you won't think about fitness. Build a new support group and a new attitude.

Keep selling yourself on fitness and health by talking about how much you enjoy exercising and its benefits. Do this for at least 6 times a day for 90 days. Enough time to develop new habits and attitudes and beliefs. If you don't, then there is up to a 95% chance of failure. If you fail to follow through, just keep trying.

Daily Log

Date_____   _____

1st-Time	Talked to:
2nd Time	Talked to:
3rd Time	Talked to:
4th Time	Talked to:
5th Time	Talked to:
6th Time	Talked to:
7th Time	Talked to:
8th Time	Talked to:
9th Time	Talked to:
10th Time	Talked to:
11th Time	Talked to:

0-595-17900-2